Herbal Remedies

A Comprehensive DIY Guide for Learning to Make Home-Made Herbal Remedies

Jeromme Maxwell

© **Copyright 2022 - All rights reserved.**

The content contained within this book may not be reproduced, duplicated or transmitted without direct written permission from the author or the publisher.

Under no circumstances will any blame or legal responsibility be held against the publisher, or author, for any damages, reparation, or monetary loss due to the information contained within this book, either directly or indirectly.

Legal Notice:

This book is copyright protected. It is only for personal use. You cannot amend, distribute, sell, use, quote or paraphrase any part, or the content within this book, without the consent of the author or publisher.

Disclaimer Notice:

Please note the information contained within this document is for educational and entertainment purposes only. All effort has been executed to present accurate, up to date, reliable, complete information. No warranties of any kind are declared or implied. Readers acknowledge that the author is not engaging in the rendering of legal, financial, medical or professional advice. The content within this book has been derived from various sources. Please consult a licensed professional before attempting any techniques outlined in this book.

By reading this document, the reader agrees that under no circumstances is the author responsible for any losses, direct or indirect, that are incurred as a result of the use of information contained within this document, including, but not limited to, errors, omissions, or inaccuracies.

Table of Contents

Introduction 1

Chapter 1: What Are Antibiotics? 4

    What Are Antibiotics? 5

    Chemical Structure of Antibiotics 5

    Bactericidal and Bacteriostatic Antibiotics 6

    Role of Antibiotics in Treatment 7

    History of Antibiotics 7

    Mode of Action of Antibiotics 8

    When to Use Antibiotics 9

    Things to Consider before Taking Antibiotics 13

    Why Is Their Use Becoming Less Common? 14

    Reasons Why People Overuse Antibiotics 15

    Why Do People Still Use Them? 15

    How Does Antibiotic Resistance Happen? 16

    Potential Drivers for Resistance 16

    What Can You Do to Prevent Antibiotic Resistance? 17

    Pros and Cons of Antibiotic Use 18

    Natural Antibiotics 20

Chapter 2: Herbal Antibiotics 22

    What Are Herbal Antibiotics? 23

How Are Herbal Antibiotics Made? 24
Herbal Antibiotics: The Most Effective Solution Against
Infections 24
Broad Spectrum Vs. Narrow Spectrum Herbal Antibiotics 25
Why Use Narrow-Spectrum Antibiotics? 26
What Makes Herbal Antibiotics So Effective? 26
Why Are Herbal Antibiotics Becoming More Popular? 27
What Are Some Common Herbal Antibiotics? 28
The Benefits of Using Herbal Antibiotics 32
How to Use Herbal Antibiotics to Treat Infections 34
Illness That Herbal Antibiotics Can Cure 34
Urinary Tract Infections 35
Bronchitis 36
Pneumonia 37
Gastrointestinal Infections 38
Skin Infections 38
Sexually Transmitted Infections 39
Blood Poisoning 40
Tuberculosis 40
Other Infections 40
Five Reasons to Keep Herbal Antibiotics in
Your Medicine Cabinet 41
How Are Herbal Antibiotics Different from
Normal Antibiotics? 42

Chapter 3: Systemic Herbal Antibiotics 44
Common Use of Systemic Herbal Antibiotic 45
Ailments Treated with Herbal Antibiotics 45

Chapter 4: Non-Systemic Herbal Antibiotics 59

What Are Non-Systemic Antibiotics? 60

Ailments Assisted by Non-Systemic Antibiotics 61

Herbs and Ingredients Used as Natural Antibiotics 64

Garlic 64

Juniper 65

Honey 67

Echinacea 68

Cranberry 68

Licorice Root 69

Olive Leaf 70

Eucalyptus 71

Ginseng 71

Shatavari 72

Shitake Mushrooms 72

Goldenseal 73

Oregano 74

Uva-ursi 75

Chapter 5: Synergist Antibiotics 77

What Does 'Synergist Antibiotics' Mean? 78

Common Use of Synergistic Antibiotics 81

Other Causes of Drug and Antibiotic Resistance 83

Natural Antibiotics 84

Chapter 6: Strengthening the Immune System 88

The Importance of Strengthening the Immune System After Using Antibiotics 89

Benefits of a Strong Immune System 90
Herbs and Ingredients That Can Be Used to
Strengthen the Immune System.. 91

Chapter 7: Herbal Medicine Making Handbook 103
Making Medicine Using Herbs... 104
Importance of Using Herbs as Medicine 105
Dangers of Using Herbs as Medicine....................................... 106
Common Ailments Around You 107
Precautions When Choosing Herbal Medicine....................... 107
Herbs for Combating Diseases 109
Tools Needed to Manage Your Herb Garden 114
Why You Should Have a Herb Garden 117
When to Avoid Herbal Medicine 118

Chapter 8: Herbal Antibiotic Recipes I 121
Do Natural Antibiotics Work?.. 122
Herbal Antibiotic Recipes to Keep You Healthy 122
Garlic, Ginger, and Turmeric Paste... 123
Echinacea Tea 125
Goldenseal Ointment 127
Echinacea Tincture 129
Oregano Oil.. 131
Rosemary Tea 133
Marshmallow Root Ointment... 135
Herbal Sore Throat Gargle 137
Lemon Balm Tea 139
Thyme Tincture.. 141

Ginger Tea 143

Hawthorn Berry Tea 145

Chapter 9: Herbal Antibiotic Recipes II 147

Peppermint Tea 147

Eucalyptus Salve 150

Rosemary and Thyme Tea 152

Wormwood Tincture 155

Chamomile Tea 157

Clove Bud Oil 159

Elderberry Tea 161

Herbal Cough Syrup 163

Herbal Throat Spray 165

Yarrow Tincture 167

Herbal Drink 169

Usnea Tincture 172

Herbal Tea for Cough Relief 174

Conclusion 176

References 179

Introduction

Since their discovery in the late 1920s, antibiotics have shaped and reshaped the history of medicine. The medicine that kills bacteria has reduced the number of people dying from common infections. This created enough excitement for pharmaceutical companies to produce it in insane amounts for a while. Doctors were encouraged to prescribe them, and people were presented with all their benefits. After all, this was the first medicine that killed bacteria without harming human cells - or so they thought. However, in the past couple of decades, it has become more than evident that synthetic antibiotics are overused. They've caused a wide range of issues even modern medicine has difficulties dealing with. During this period, the focus shifted to the production and use of natural antibiotics - the topic of this book.

Plants have been used in natural medicine for thousands of years. Ancient remedies were prepared for a plethora of conditions, including infections. With the development of the modern sciences, many bioactive compounds in herbs have been isolated. Their actions have been thoroughly studied, allowing us to understand how they benefit the body. Due to this, we know that herbal antibiotics act on the same principle as their synthetic counterparts; they kill the bacteria spreading throughout the body.

The difference is that herbal antibiotics also help the body to recover. You don't need months of prebiotic treatments after using herbal antibiotics. The combination of herbs is often devised so that it sheds the cells from getting damaged during the treatment. While, in challenging cases, the additional use of natural healing agents is still necessary, herbal antibiotics protect the immune system instead of weakening it.

The emergence of antibiotic-resistant bacteria is a compelling reason to switch to natural antibiotics. However, there are several more. Some additional therapeutic effects of herb-based or herb-derived antibiotics include a stronger immune system and a healthier liver and kidney metabolism. All these justify the use of herbs for healing infections and diseases. You'll read more about how herbal antibiotics act compared to synthetic drugs in the first few chapters of this book.

You'll be introduced to the main herbal antivirals and learn which plants and combinations of plants can be used for each purpose. Knowing how each herbal ingredient acts is crucial for determining the appropriate course of treatment, even with natural medicine. It's best to grow your own herb garden and build an herb lab where you prepare the medicine to ensure the plants act as they should. It means investing in different tools and equipment, but it's an investment that'll definitely pay off. You won't have to pay for artificial medicine or different herbal ingredients when you need them.

Besides learning about the effects of plants and their possible combinations, it's also crucial to use the right ingredient quantities. Fortunately, this book provides plenty of beginner-friendly recipes for preparing herbal antibiotics. Following them is highly recommended to avoid mistakes, especially if you're learning. So, if you're ready to begin your journey of learning to treat infections and illnesses naturally, all you need to do is read this book.

Chapter 1

What Are Antibiotics?

Antibiotics treat various bacterial infections and can be very effective for improving your health when used correctly. Your doctor normally prescribes antibiotics when you get sick. These drugs fight bacteria to help you recover faster. But what are antibiotics? They are common medicines that fight bacteria by stopping their growth.

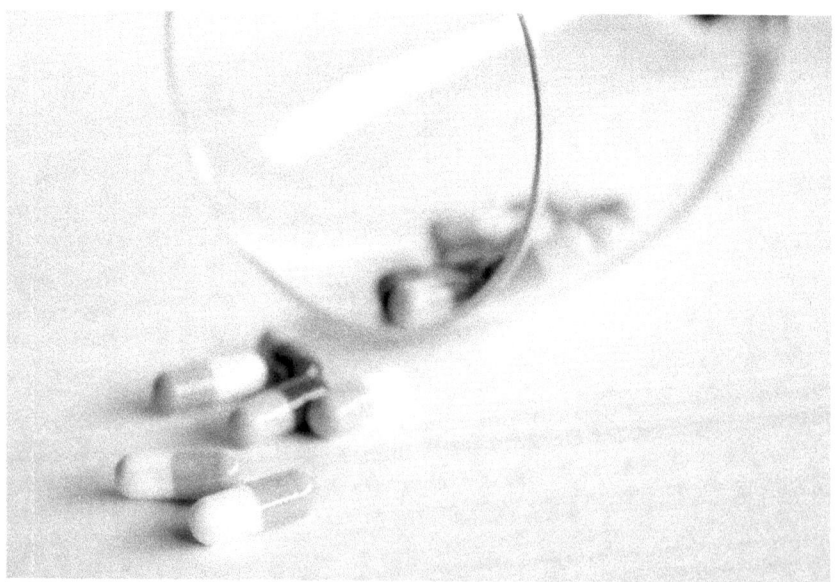

Unfortunately, the overuse of antibiotics leads to resistance in some bacteria strains, making them tougher to treat the next time. This book covers everything about antibiotics — what they are, how they work, and how to use them responsibly to continue working effectively in the future.

What Are Antibiotics?

Antibiotics are medications used to treat infections caused by bacteria. They work by killing the bacteria or preventing them from growing. Antibiotics are usually only prescribed for bacterial infections, as they are ineffective against viruses. There are many different antibiotics, each targeting different bacteria, meaning that an antibiotic can treat almost any bacterial infection.

Some common antibiotics include amoxicillin, ciprofloxacin, and erythromycin. Antibiotics are usually taken for 7-10 days. Despite feeling better after a few days, finishing the entire antibiotic course is essential because stopping the medication early allows the bacteria to grow and the infection to return. It can also lead to antibiotic resistance, which is discussed later.

Chemical Structure of Antibiotics

Antibiotics are usually small molecules with a specific chemical structure. This chemical structure helps them bind to bacterial cells and kill or prevent them from growing. The most common antibiotic is the beta-lactam antibiotic. Beta-lactam antibiotics work by binding to a protein called penicillin-binding proteins (PBPs).

PBPs are found in the bacterial cell wall and help hold it together. Beta-lactam antibiotics bind to PBPs and prevent the bacteria from building or repairing cell walls, eventually leading to the bacteria's death.

Other antibiotics work differently. For example, tetracyclines bind to the bacterial ribosome (the part of the cell that makes proteins), preventing the bacteria from making new proteins, eventually leading to the bacteria's death.

Other antibiotics work differently, but the overall goal is to kill or prevent bacteria growth.

Bactericidal and Bacteriostatic Antibiotics

Antibiotics can be broadly divided into two groups: bactericidal and bacteriostatic. Bactericidal antibiotics kill bacteria, while bacteriostatic antibiotics prevent bacteria growth. Bactericidal antibiotics are generally more effective than bacteriostatic antibiotics, providing a quicker and more complete cure. However, both ways can treat a bacterial infection effectively.

All antibiotics must undergo clinical trials before they can be prescribed as part of a treatment plan. These trials determine how safe and effective the antibiotics are. Depending on your infection, your doctor will prescribe you a specific antibiotic.

For antibiotics to work effectively, they must reach the body part where bacteria have developed. This happens in three ways:

Systemic Antibiotics: These are taken by mouth or given as an injection and travel through the bloodstream to reach the infection.

Topical Antibiotics: These are applied directly to the skin or an eye, ear, or wound.

Local Antibiotics: These are injected directly into a body cavity, joint, or tissue.

Role of Antibiotics in Treatment

Antibiotics are essential in treating bacterial infections. They can help cure the disease and improve your overall health. In some cases, antibiotics are the only treatment option available. This is especially true in severe infections, such as pneumonia or meningitis.

In other cases, antibiotics are used alongside other treatments. For example, you will be prescribed antibiotics and antiviral medication if you simultaneously have bacterial and viral infections. Antibiotics are not always the answer to treating a bacterial infection. In some cases, they do more harm than good.

History of Antibiotics

The first antibiotic was penicillin, discovered in 1928 by Scottish scientist Alexander Fleming. Fleming's discovery was accidental. He was investigating a group of bacteria called staphylococci, and he noticed that one of the plates he was using had been contaminated with a mold called Penicillium. The mold killed the bacteria, and Fleming realized he had discovered a substance that could kill bacteria without harming humans.

In the early days of antibiotic development, penicillin was used to treat human wounds. It was successful in many cases, and the US government supported the mass production of penicillin. By World War II, penicillin had become known as "the wonder drug" for its success in treating infections. Scientists in Oxford were crucial in developing the mass production process for penicillin and were recognized with a Nobel Prize in 1945.

In the 1980s, health organizations worldwide began warning people about the overuse of antibiotics. Over time, bacteria have evolved and developed a resistance to antibiotics, causing many common infections to become harder to treat. This could lead to a health crisis if we don't find a way to stop bacteria from becoming immune to antibiotics.

Mode of Action of Antibiotics

The mode of action of an antibiotic is how it kills or prevents the growth of bacteria.

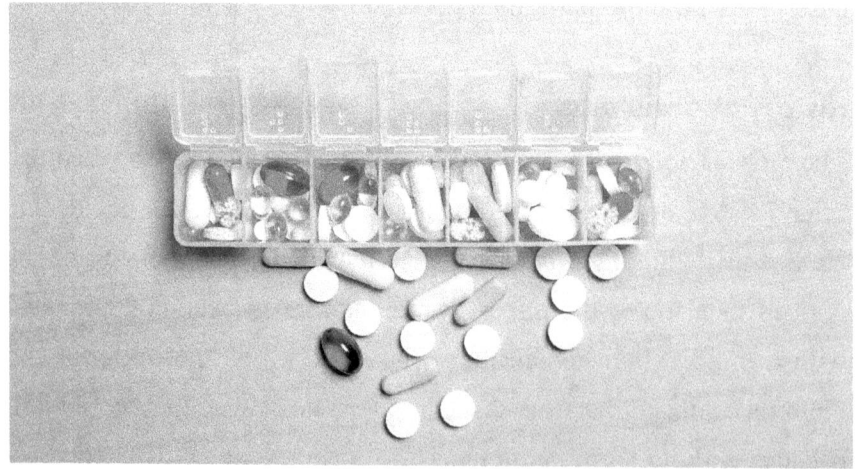

Different antibiotics work differently. Some antibiotics kill bacteria by preventing them from building their cell walls, while others prevent them from making new proteins.

Different antibiotics also work on different parts of the bacteria. Some antibiotics target the bacteria's cell wall, and others target the proteins the bacteria use to reproduce.

Finally, some antibiotics work by disrupting how the bacteria communicate with each other. This communication is necessary for the bacteria to coordinate their activities and are essential to causing disease.

The mode of action of an antibiotic is an essential factor in choosing the right antibiotic for a particular infection. For example, if a condition is caused by bacteria resistant to one antibiotic, a different antibiotic with a different mode of action can be effective.

Antibiotics work by targeting specific bacteria, meaning they are only effective against the bacteria they are designed to target. They will not kill viruses, and they will not kill healthy bacteria.

When to Use Antibiotics

If you have a bacterial infection, taking antibiotics can speed up your recovery. But there are times when they're not the best choice. You could be prescribed antibiotics if you have any of the following conditions:

Ear Infections

Ear infections can range from mild to severe. Most ear infections are caused by bacteria and are treated with antibiotics. Antibiotics are suggested for severe ear infections that are caused by bacteria.

Your doctor will likely prescribe antibiotics if you have an ear infection. But in some cases, ear infections go away on their own within a few days. So, your doctor should wait to see if the infection goes away before prescribing antibiotics.

The same is true for sinus infections and bronchitis. These illnesses are often caused by viruses, which don't respond to antibiotics.

Respiratory Tract Infections

The common cold, sorest throats, and bronchitis are all caused by viruses. These illnesses usually go away on their own within a week or two. Taking antibiotics won't help you get better any faster or cause side effects.

However, you need antibiotics if you have a bacterial infection, like strep throat or tonsillitis. These infections are usually diagnosed with a throat swab.

Urinary Tract Infections

A urinary tract infection (UTI) is an infection in any part of your urinary system — your kidneys, ureters, bladder, and urethra.

Most UTIs are caused by bacteria, such as Escherichia coli, Klebsiella pneumonia, or Staphylococcus saprophyticus. A UTI can also be caused by a virus, like the one that causes the common cold or flu.

UTIs occur more often in women than men because the urethra — the tube that carries urine from the bladder to the outside body — is shorter in women than in men. Therefore, it is easier for bacteria to travel from the outside of the body to the bladder.

UTIs are also more common in older adults. The aging process weakens the muscles in the bladder and causes changes in the lining of the urinary tract, making it easier for bacteria to grow.

Most UTIs can be treated with antibiotics. But sometimes, they go away on their own; this is more likely to happen if the UTI is in the lower urinary tract — the urethra and bladder.

Sinus Infection

Viruses or bacteria can cause sinus infections. Antibiotics are only effective against bacteria. Therefore, if your sinus infection is caused by a virus, taking antibiotics will not help or do more harm than good. However, if your sinus infection is caused by bacteria, taking antibiotics will help to clear the infection.

Skin Infections

Skin infections are often caused by staphylococcus or streptococcus bacteria. Antibiotics can help treat these infections. Some common skin infections that antibiotics can treat are:

Cellulitis: This is a bacterial infection of the skin and underlying tissues. It often affects the legs but can occur anywhere on the body.

Impetigo: This is a contagious bacterial skin infection. It causes sores and blisters.

Folliculitis: This is an infection of the hair follicles. It can cause pus-filled bumps on the skin.

Antibiotics can also be used to treat acne. However, they are not always effective and can have side effects.

Infected Wounds

Wounds can become infected with bacteria, for instance, after an injury or surgery. Infected wounds can be painful, cause swelling, and lead to serious complications.

Your doctor prescribes antibiotics to treat an infected wound to help kill the bacteria and prevent the infection from spreading.

See your doctor if you think you have an infection. They will diagnose the infection and prescribe the appropriate treatment. In some cases, home remedies are all that you need. But in other cases, you will need antibiotics.

Don't treat an infection yourself with over-the-counter medication; this could worsen the infection. Also, it is essential not to take antibiotics prescribed for someone else. It could delay the treatment and increase your risk of complications.

Pneumonia

Pneumonia is a serious lung infection. Bacteria, viruses, or fungi can cause it.

The most common cause of pneumonia in adults is bacteria called Streptococcus pneumonia (sometimes called pneumococcus). Other bacteria that because pneumonia include Haemophilus influenza and Mycoplasma pneumonia.

Viral causes of pneumonia include influenza (flu) and respiratory syncytial virus (RSV). These viruses are the most common cause of pneumonia in children.

Fungal pneumonia is rare. The most common type is caused by fungi called Pneumocystis jirovecii. It usually only affects people with weakened immune systems, such as HIV/AIDS, cancer, or organ transplant recipients.

Antibiotics are not effective against viral or fungal pneumonia. However, they can be prescribed if you have a bacterial infection and your lungs are also infected with a virus or fungi. The bacteria make the viral or fungal infection worse.

Things to Consider before Taking Antibiotics

It's essential only to accept antibiotics when necessary. Ask your doctor if you have any questions about whether or not you should take an antibiotic. It is necessary to take antibiotics exactly as your doctor prescribes; this means completing the entire course of antibiotics, even if you feel better.

Second, taking antibiotics can lead to antibiotic resistance. In this case, bacteria become resistant to antibiotics. When this happens, the antibiotic becomes less effective against that particular bacteria.

Finally, taking antibiotics can have side effects. These side effects could range from mild to severe, including nausea, vomiting, diarrhea, and rashes. If you experience severe side effects, you must immediately stop taking antibiotics and seek medical help.

Why Is Their Use Becoming Less Common?

Antibiotics are becoming less common because bacteria are becoming more resistant. The excessive use of antibiotics is causing bacteria to become immune to the medication. When people take antibiotics, the bacteria in their bodies are exposed to the drug. Some bacteria die, but some survive and multiply. These surviving bacteria are now resistant to the antibiotic and can pass this resistance on to their offspring.

The World Health Organization has reported that this growing antibiotic resistance is one of today's most significant global health threats. As bacteria become more resistant to antibiotics, the drugs become less effective. It is a significant problem. We are running out of options for treating bacterial infections, so antibiotics aren't as effective as they once were.

Antibiotics treat specific bacterial infections, like ear infections or UTIs. Antibiotics are not designed to treat common cold or flu viral infections. Using antibiotics to treat viral infections is ineffective and can cause more harm to your body. If you feel unwell and think you need antibiotics, your doctor will need to run tests to rule out a viral infection first. Taking antibiotics when you don't need them can lead to antibiotic resistance.

Reasons Why People Overuse Antibiotics

One reason is that many people do not finish their entire antibiotics course. They feel better after a few days and think they do not need to take the rest of the pills. The bacteria might not be killed entirely if the course is not completed. As a result, the bacteria can become resistant to the antibiotic.

Another reason for the overuse of antibiotics is that they are often prescribed unnecessarily. For example, many viral infections cannot be treated with antibiotics. However, many doctors prescribe them anyway because patients expect to receive them.

The overuse of antibiotics is a significant problem because it leads to antibiotic resistance - when bacteria become resistant to the effects of antibiotics. As a result, more and more infections are becoming difficult or impossible to treat.

Why Do People Still Use Them?

Even though the overuse of antibiotics is causing bacteria to become resistant, people still use them. One reason is that people don't know whether they have a bacterial or viral infection. They often think they need antibiotics when they don't.

Another reason people continue to use antibiotics is that they expect to feel better immediately. You must wait a few days with most medications to see results; this isn't the case with antibiotics. When people take antibiotics, they usually feel better within a day or two.

People also use antibiotics because they think they will prevent future infections. Antibiotics help prevent infections if you have been exposed to bacteria. But they won't help you to avoid getting sick in the future.

How Does Antibiotic Resistance Happen?

Antibiotic resistance occurs when bacteria mutate and develop a resistance to the medication. When this happens, the antibiotic is no longer effective in treating the infection.

Bacteria can become resistant to antibiotics in several ways. One way is by random mutation; this is a natural process that happens over time. As the bacteria multiply, they sometimes mutate and develop resistance to the antibiotic.

Another way bacteria can become resistant is by sharing genetic material with other bacteria; this happens when the bacteria are exposed to the antibiotic. Some bacteria will die, but some will survive and multiply. Bacteria that survive and reproduce now possess resistance to the antibiotic. Increasingly resistant bacteria make antibiotics less effective.

Potential Drivers for Resistance

Many potential drivers are for antibiotic resistance. One of the main drivers is the overuse and misuse of antibiotics. When antibiotics are used too often, or for the wrong reasons, it can cause bacteria to become resistant.

Antibiotics are commonly used in livestock, which can contribute to the problem of antibiotic resistance. Farmers often give animals low antibiotic doses to prevent them from getting sick. However, this practice can also lead to the development of antibiotic-resistant bacteria. These bacteria can be passed on to humans through the food supply.

Another potential driver for antibiotic resistance is using broad-spectrum antibiotics. These drugs are designed to kill a wide range of bacteria. However, they can also kill the good bacteria in our bodies, allowing antibiotic-resistant bacteria to take over.

The overuse of antibiotics in healthcare is also a potential driver for antibiotic resistance. In some cases, patients pressure their doctors to prescribe antibiotics when they are not necessary. In other cases, doctors prescribe antibiotics as a precautionary measure, even when unsure if the patient has a bacterial infection.

All these factors contribute to the development of antibiotic-resistant bacteria. Therefore, bacterial infections are becoming increasingly difficult to treat.

What Can You Do to Prevent Antibiotic Resistance?

It's important to remember that antibiotic resistance is a natural phenomenon. It's not something we can eliminate. However, we can reduce the rate at which bacteria become resistant to antibiotics.

One way is by reducing the unnecessary use of antibiotics. Antibiotics should only be used to treat bacterial infections. They should not be used to treat viral infections like the flu.

Only take antibiotics when a doctor prescribes them. If you are prescribed antibiotics, you must take them exactly as directed. Do not skip doses, and do not stop taking the medication early.

It is also essential to finish all your prescribed medications, even if you feel better; this will help ensure that all the bacteria are killed.

If you have leftover antibiotics, do not save them for later. Throw them away according to the instructions on the label.

You can also help to prevent antibiotic resistance by washing your hands regularly and cooking meat thoroughly. These measures will help to reduce your exposure to bacteria.

Antibiotic resistance is a significant problem today. Antibiotics can remain effective for years if we prevent them from occurring.

Pros and Cons of Antibiotic Use

Antibiotics are drugs that treat bacterial infections. Antibiotics can be very effective in treating these conditions but have some potential drawbacks.

One of the main advantages of using antibiotics is that they can help clear an infection quickly. It is especially important for illnesses that could potentially be serious or life-threatening. Antibiotics can also prevent infections from occurring in the first place. For example, they can be given before surgery to prevent disease.

However, there are also some disadvantages to using antibiotics. Antibiotics' most common side effects are stomach upset, diarrhea, and nausea, but they usually go away after a few days. You must seek medical attention immediately if you experience severe side effects, like a rash or difficulty breathing.

Some people are allergic to certain antibiotics. An allergic reaction must be treated immediately, such as a rash, hives, or difficulty breathing.

Antibiotics can also interact with other medications. You must inform your doctor about all your medicines, including over-the-counter drugs, vitamins, and herbal supplements.

Additionally, overuse of antibiotics can sometimes lead to antibiotic resistance. The bacteria become more resistant to the effects of these drugs; this makes it more difficult to treat infections in the future.

Another potential disadvantage of using antibiotics is that they can kill good bacteria. It can lead to an imbalance in the body's natural bacteria, making a person more susceptible to other infections. Additionally, when good bacteria are killed, it allows harmful bacteria to thrive and potentially cause more harm.

Overall, there are both advantages and disadvantages to using antibiotics. It is important to weigh these factors when deciding whether or not to use these drugs. Additionally, it is crucial to follow the directions of a healthcare provider when taking antibiotics and to finish the entire treatment course, even if symptoms improve, to prevent resistance and further complications.

Natural Antibiotics

In recent years, there has been a growing interest in natural antibiotics. These are substances occurring naturally in the environment and have antibacterial properties.

Several natural antibiotics can treat bacterial infections. These include garlic, honey, and oregano oil.

Garlic has antibacterial, antiviral, and antifungal properties. It works by inhibiting bacteria growth. Honey is another popular natural antibiotic. It has been used to treat wounds and burns for centuries. Oregano oil is an essential oil with antibacterial, antifungal, and antiviral properties.

Natural antibiotics are generally considered safe and well-tolerated. When using natural antibiotics, it is essential to remember that they are not as strong as traditional antibiotics, meaning they are ineffective against all bacteria. It's essential to speak with your doctor before using any natural remedy, as they can interact with other medications you're taking.

Although antibiotics have been around for quite some time, there is still much we do not know about them – including the potential dangers of antibiotic overuse. It is essential to take any medication as directed by your doctor and finish all the prescribed doses.

Remember, merely because an antibiotic is available over-the-counter does not mean it is safe to take without consulting a physician first.

Chapter 2

Herbal Antibiotics

With the rise of antibiotic-resistant bacteria, many people look for natural alternatives to traditional medicine. Herbal antibiotics are one option gaining popularity. Herbal antibiotics are natural substances with antimicrobial activity against bacteria. Generally, these can be obtained from plants, fruits, and other vegetable sources.

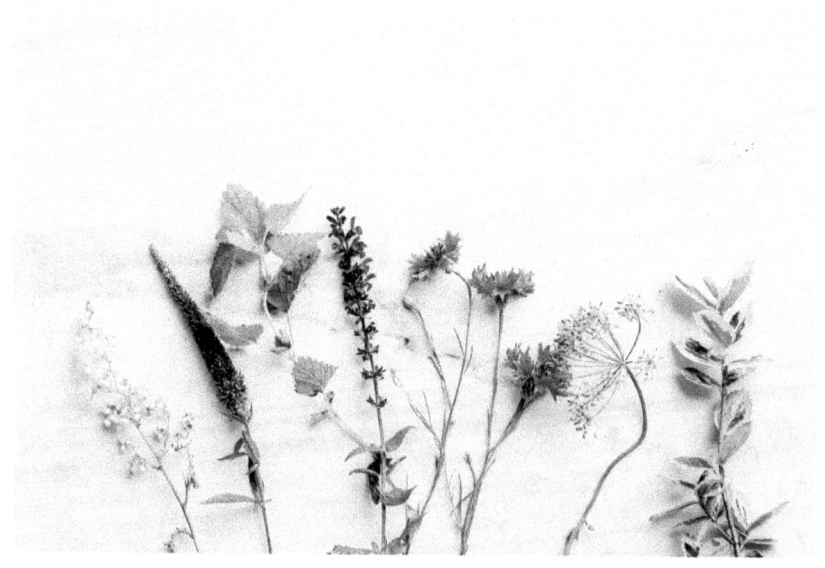

They usually have low toxicity and have been used for centuries to treat human diseases. However, there is no universal list of herbal antibiotics; each plant has its compounds with specific properties and actions on pathogens, so their use must be evaluated individually for each case.

What Are Herbal Antibiotics?

An antibiotic is a substance that inhibits the growth of, or kills, bacteria. More specifically, it is any substance produced by a microorganism that inhibits the growth of other organisms in the same species.

Herbal antibiotics are antimicrobial herbs that help fight infections by killing bacteria or inhibiting their growth. They have been used for centuries in traditional medicine to treat various illnesses, including bronchitis, sinus infections, and urinary tract infections. Herbal antibiotics are becoming more popular as people look for alternatives to conventional antibiotics, which have side effects such as gastrointestinal upset, skin rashes, and yeast infections.

Herbal antibiotics work on bacteria differently. The exact mechanism of action of herbal antibiotics is not fully understood. Since their precise mode of action is unknown, it is difficult to predict their effect on bacteria strains that develop resistance.

Some herbal antibiotics disrupt the bacterial cell wall, and others inhibit bacterial growth by disrupting the bacterial ribosome's function. Still, others inhibit bacterial DNA replication or transcription. Some herbal antibiotics are also affected by disturbing bacterial metabolic pathways.

For example, some herbs, like oregano, have antimicrobial properties that help fight infections by destroying the bacteria. Other herbs, like garlic, act as natural antibiotic agents by inhibiting the bacteria's growth.

How Are Herbal Antibiotics Made?

Herbal antibiotics comprise complex compounds allowing them to target and destroy the harmful bacteria in an infection while leaving the good bacteria intact. The compounds in herbal antibiotics are much more difficult for harmful bacteria to break down and resist.

The active ingredients in herbal antibiotics are phytochemicals and plant-derived chemicals with antimicrobial activity. These phytochemicals can be extracted from the plant through distillation or maceration. The extract is concentrated into a tincture, capsule, or cream.

Herbal Antibiotics: The Most Effective Solution Against Infections

Bacteria are everywhere. They exist on our skin, in the air, and in our gut. While most bacteria are harmless, some cause infections. These infections can range from mild to life-threatening.

The first line of defense against these harmful bacteria is our immune system. However, sometimes the bacteria are too strong, and our immune system can't fight them off; this is when we need antibiotics.

While antibiotics are generally safe and effective, they can have side effects. In addition, some bacteria are becoming resistant to antibiotics, meaning the antibiotics will not work against these bacteria.

Herbal antibiotics are a possible solution to this problem. Infections can be treated with herbal antibiotics because they are made from plants and other natural substances. Therefore, they are immensely beneficial to our body's health. When we suffer from a disease, our immune system cannot fight it on its own, which will lead to a higher risk of developing more infections and illnesses due to fighting the initial infection.

Herbal antibiotics are generally safe and have few side effects. They are also effective against bacteria resistant to antibiotics.

Broad Spectrum Vs. Narrow Spectrum Herbal Antibiotics

There are two main herbal antibiotics: broad spectrum and narrow spectrum. A broad-spectrum antibiotic is effective against gram-positive and gram-negative bacteria. A narrow-spectrum antibiotic is effective only against one bacteria type.

The main difference between the two antibiotic types is that broad-spectrum antibiotics are effective against a broader range of bacteria. In contrast, narrow-spectrum antibiotics are only effective against specific bacteria. For example, your doctor can prescribe a narrow-spectrum antibiotic to kill Streptococcus bacteria if you have a strep throat infection.

Narrow-spectrum antibiotics are sometimes used when a patient is allergic to a broad-spectrum antibiotic. For example, suppose you are allergic to penicillin. A narrow-spectrum antibiotic can be prescribed to treat your infection without causing an allergic reaction.

Broad-spectrum herbal antibiotics prevent infections in people at risk of developing an infection. For example, suppose you have a urinary tract infection caused by gram-positive and gram-negative bacteria - your doctor can prescribe a broad-spectrum antibiotic like ciprofloxacin.

Why Use Narrow-Spectrum Antibiotics?

Narrow spectrum antibiotics are effective against specific bacteria strains. They destroy the bacteria's cell wall, preventing it from rebuilding and causing it to die. It is advantageous because it targets explicitly harmful bacteria without harming good bacteria. Additionally, it minimizes the chances of developing antibiotic resistance.

The antibiotic that is right for you depends on your infection. Your doctor will determine the best treatment based on your medical history and the severity of your condition.

What Makes Herbal Antibiotics So Effective?

Herbal antibiotics have been used for centuries to treat a variety of infections. In recent years, there has been a resurgence in interest in these natural remedies as more and more people look for alternatives to conventional antibiotics.

The complexity of the compounds in herbal antibiotics is what makes them so effective. Harmful bacteria have difficulty breaking down these complex compounds, but herbal antibiotics can easily break down and resist the harmful bacteria. It is mainly due to the metabolism process; this is much more difficult in pharmaceutical antibiotics because they only possess one potent compound.

Herbal antibiotics are more effective than synthetic ones for many reasons. For one, they are more targeted in their action and less likely to cause collateral damage to beneficial gut flora with broad-spectrum antibiotics.

They are also gentler on the body, causing fewer side effects. Since they are derived from natural sources, they are less likely to contribute to the development of antibiotic resistance.

Herbal antibiotics are an excellent choice for those wanting a natural and effective way to fight infection.

Why Are Herbal Antibiotics Becoming More Popular?

The emergence of antibiotic resistance has made it necessary to explore alternative methods to combat bacterial infections. Using herbal antibiotics to treat infections caused by bacteria has been around for centuries.

Herbal antibiotics have fewer side effects and are an alternative to synthetic antibiotics to treat bacterial infections. Unlike synthetic antibiotics, which can kill good and bad bacteria, herbal antibiotics target only bad bacteria, reducing the risk of developing antibiotic resistance.

What Are Some Common Herbal Antibiotics?

Goldenseal

Goldenseal is a perennial herb native to North America. The plant's root and rhizome (underground stem) are used to make medicine. Goldenseal is commonly used as an antimicrobial and anti-inflammatory. It is effective in treating respiratory infections, urinary tract infections, and gastrointestinal infections.

Echinacea

Echinacea is a flower native to North America. The flower has a long history with Native Americans for its medicinal properties. Echinacea is most commonly used to boost the immune system and help fight infections. The flower also has anti-inflammatory and pain-relieving properties.

Ginger

Ginger is one of the best herbal antibiotics. It's especially effective against stomach, respiratory, and skin infections. The active ingredients in ginger are particularly good at fighting bacteria, making it a beneficial herbal antibiotic.

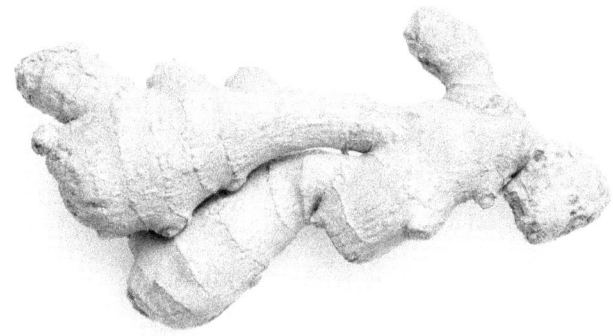

One downside to ginger is that it is heat-sensitive, so it's best to take it in capsule form, raw, or as a very light mixture. However, this shouldn't stop you from enjoying your favorite foods – ginger can enhance the flavor of many dishes. However, be careful not to neutralize its antibacterial properties when cooking. You can use ginger as a delicious and effective herbal antibiotic with care.

Aloe Vera

Aloe Vera is succulent, meaning it retains water well. The plant is most commonly known for treating minor burns from the sun or a kitchen accident. The gel found in Aloe Vera can treat cold sores, cuts, and scrapes.

However, aloe vera also has antibacterial and antifungal properties, making it helpful in treating other skin conditions, such as eczema, psoriasis, and acne. Aloe vera can also be taken internally to treat digestive issues.

Mint Family

Different plants in the mint family can be used as culinary herbs with antibiotic properties - oregano, thyme, basil, peppermint, lavender, and spearmint are a few. The unique taste of mints is what makes them effective against infection. Chemicals and oils in the characteristic taste have antimicrobial properties. To use mints, add them to vegetable soup - colds and flu infections respond well to this remedy.

Mint family herbs, including elderberries and licorice, are effective against colds and flu. Elderberries protect the body against influenza viruses and shorten the duration of the illness, while licorice strengthens the immune system. Those with kidney-related diseases or high blood pressure should avoid these herbs.

Eucalyptus

Eucalyptus is most effectively used against respiratory infections but can also be used for other illnesses. It is an herb that can fight bacterial infections. It is best used when added to a pot of boiling water for fifteen to twenty minutes, and the vapors are inhaled.

Some precautions should be taken when using eucalyptus, like avoiding inhalation if you have asthma or other respiratory problems. You should also avoid taking eucalyptus internally.

Croton Latex

Croton latex is a powerful herbal antibiotic from the sap of a tree in the Amazon rainforest. It is most effective when applied to external wounds, like cuts and burns. Croton latex also has the added benefit of protecting against further infection by creating a seal over the wound. It is especially important for external damages, as they are more susceptible to disease. Croton latex can be applied directly to the skin or taken orally.

Croton latex can cause allergic reactions in people. If you experience any symptoms of an allergic reaction, such as rash, itching, or swelling, stop using croton latex and see your doctor. Pregnant and breastfeeding women should avoid using croton latex.

Olive Leaf

Olive leaf is traditionally used for its medicinal properties, including broad-spectrum antibacterial activity and anti-viral, antifungal, and anti-inflammatory properties. These characteristics make olive leaf an effective natural remedy for various respiratory, candida, and staphylococcus infections. Olive leaf is a bronchodilator and general immune tonic, making it an effective preventative measure against respiratory tract infections.

Olive leaf extract can be taken as a capsule or liquid extract. It can also be applied topically to the skin. Some people experience side effects such as diarrhea, nausea, and headaches when taking olive leaf extract. If you experience any side effects, stop taking the supplement and consult your doctor.

Herbal Teas

Herbal teas, particularly those made with tea tree leaves, can be effective against harmful bacteria. Tea tree oil is especially lethal to yeast and staph bacteria and helps prevent bacteria growth on the skin and nose.

Tea is most effective when used twice a day for six months. In some cases, tea completely cures the infection. However, there are some disadvantages to using tea as an antibiotic.

Similarly, tea tree oil can cause skin irritation and should only be used externally. Tea should also not be taken internally.

The Benefits of Using Herbal Antibiotics

The use of herbal medicines has been on the rise recently as people look for more naturalistic and holistic approaches to their health. Herbal antibiotics can treat infections caused by multiple bacterial species resistant to synthetic antibiotics.

Herbal antibiotics have bactericidal, bacteriostatic, and disinfectant properties, used for different conditions. Herbal antibiotics can be applied locally for topical infections, eye infections, and intravenously for severe systemic diseases.

Herbal antibiotics are effective against many bacteria, including gram-positive and gram-negative strains, which can treat various bacterial and viral infections. Herbal antibiotics are one area where herbs can be extremely helpful, and many different benefits come from using them.

Herbal Antibiotics Are Safe

One of the biggest benefits of using herbal antibiotics is that they are much safer than traditional antibiotics because herbs don't create the same side effects as pharmaceutical ones. Herbal antibiotics are less likely to create resistant bacteria strains, which is a major problem with traditional antibiotics.

Herbal Antibiotics Are Natural

Another benefit of using herbal antibiotics is that they are completely natural. They will not interact with any other medications, and they will not have any negative side effects.

Herbal antibiotics are generally much gentler on the body than conventional antibiotics because they work with the body's natural systems rather than fighting against them. As a result, herbal antibiotics are often much better tolerated by the body and cause fewer side effects.

Herbal Antibiotics Are Affordable

One of the biggest benefits of using herbal antibiotics is that they are much cheaper than traditional antibiotics. Herbs are inexpensive to grow and harvest and can be easily sourced from many places. In addition, herbal antibiotics don't require a prescription, so you can save even more money by avoiding doctor's visits.

Herbal Antibiotics Are Effective

Although they are natural, herbal antibiotics are quite effective because they contain powerful compounds that kill bacteria and viruses. Some herbal antibiotics are as effective as traditional antibiotics and can treat various infections.

While herbal antibiotics are not right for everyone, they can be a great option for those wanting a more naturalistic approach to their health. If you are considering using herbal antibiotics, you must talk to your doctor to ensure they are right for you.

How to Use Herbal Antibiotics to Treat Infections

Herbal antibiotics are most effective when combined with other herbs. It allows the herbal antibiotics to work synergistically, meaning the overall effect is greater than the sum of the individual products. For example, combining an herb with antibacterial properties with an herb that boosts the immune system is more effective than using either herb alone.

Choosing the right herbs for the specific infection is essential when using herbal antibiotics. Different herbs have different mechanisms of action and can be more or less effective against various bacteria. For example, some herbs are more effective against gram-positive bacteria and others against gram-negative bacteria. It is also essential to consider the severity of the infection when choosing herbal antibiotics. For more severe conditions, combining different herbs or higher doses of the herb is necessary.

Illness That Herbal Antibiotics Can Cure

Herbal antibiotics are effective against many infections, including those resistant to conventional antibiotics. Herbal antibiotics are often more potent than their synthetic counterparts and have fewer side effects.

Many different herbs can be used as antibiotics. Some of the most common include:

- Goldenseal (Hydrastis canadensis)
- Echinacea (Echinacea purpurea)
- Garlic (Allium sativum)
- Ginger (Zingiber officinale)

These herbs can be taken internally or externally (for example, as a compress). They are used in various forms, such as tinctures, teas, capsules, or powders.

Herbal antibiotics are most effective when used at the first sign of infection. However, they can treat more serious infections. If you suspect an infection, it is important to see a healthcare provider to get a proper diagnosis and treatment.

Some illnesses that herbal antibiotics can cure include:

Urinary Tract Infections

Urinary tract infections (UTIs) are one of the most common infections caused by bacteria that enter the urinary tract. UTIs affect the bladder, urethra, or kidneys.

Symptoms Of UTI Include

- Burning sensation when urinating

- Frequent urination
- Urgent need to urinate
- Cloudy or bloody urine
- Pain in the lower abdomen or back

UTIs can lead to kidney damage and other serious health problems if left untreated.

Herbal antibiotics that can treat UTIs include:

- Goldenseal
- Uva ursi (Arctostaphylos uva-ursi)
- Cranberry (Vaccinium macrocarpon)

Bronchitis

Bronchitis is an inflammation of the airways. It is usually caused by a viral infection but can also be caused by bacteria or irritants.

Symptoms of Bronchitis Include

- Coughing
- Sore throat
- Wheezing
- Shortness of breath
- Chest pain
- Fever
- Fatigue

Herbal antibiotics that can treat bronchitis include:

- Thyme (Thymus vulgaris)
- Oregano (Origanum vulgare)
- Marshmallow (Althaea officinalis)

Pneumonia

Pneumonia is a serious lung infection. Viruses, bacteria, or fungi can cause it.

Symptoms of Pneumonia Include

- Cough with phlegm
- Shortness of breath
- Chest pain
- Fever
- Sweating and chills
- Nausea and vomiting

Herbal antibiotics that can treat pneumonia include:

- Lungwort (Pulmonaria officinalis)
- Horseradish (Armoracia rusticana)
- Olive leaf (Olea europaea)

Gastrointestinal Infections

Gastrointestinal infections are another common illness effectively treated with herbal antibiotics. These infections are typically caused by a virus, bacteria, or parasite and can lead to the following symptoms:

- Diarrhea
- Nausea
- Vomiting
- Abdominal pain
- Fever

Herbal antibiotics that can treat gastrointestinal infections include:

- Chamomile (Matricaria chamomilla)
- Ginger (Zingiber officinale)
- Peppermint (Mentha piperita)

Skin Infections

Another common infection is a skin infection caused by several factors, including bacteria, viruses, and fungi. Skin infections are usually treatable with over-the-counter (OTC) medications, but more severe infections require antibiotics. Herbal antibiotics are effective in treating skin infections.

Symptoms of a Skin Infection Include

- Redness

- Swelling
- Pain
- Pus or drainage from the site
- Fever

Herbal antibiotics that can treat skin infections include:

- Calendula (Calendula officinalis)
- Echinacea (Echinacea purpurea)
- Tea tree oil (Melaleuca alternifolia)

Sexually Transmitted Infections

Bacteria, viruses, or parasites cause sexually transmitted infections (STIs). They can be passed from person to person during sexual contact. STIs cause a range of symptoms, including no symptoms at all. Some STIs lead to serious health problems, including infertility and even death.

Symptoms of an STI Include

- Sores or bumps in the genital or anal area
- Discharge from the penis or vagina
- Burning sensation when urinating
- Itching or burning in the genital area
- Painful intercourse

Herbal antibiotics that can treat STIs include:

- Garlic (Allium sativum)
- Green tea (Camellia sinensis)
- Honey

Blood Poisoning

Blood poisoning, known as septicemia, is a potentially life-threatening infection that occurs when bacteria enter the bloodstream. Herbal antibiotics used to treat blood poisoning include garlic, usnea, and echinacea.

Tuberculosis

Tuberculosis is a bacterial infection most often affecting the lungs. The best herbs and antibiotics against tuberculosis include garlic, red clovers, usnea, goldenseal, elecampane, and boneset.

Other Infections

Herbal antibiotics are also effective against other infections, including gonorrhea, tonsillitis, and bacteremia. They can also be effective against superficial infected wounds.

Some of the most common illnesses can be treated with herbal antibiotics. While herbal antibiotics are generally safe and effective, understanding that herbal antibiotics are not appropriate for everyone is crucial. For example, pregnant or breastfeeding women should not use them. People with certain medical conditions, like kidney disease, should avoid using them.

If you consider using herbal antibiotics, it is important to consult with a healthcare provider knowledgeable about herbs and their uses. It will ensure you use the right herb for your condition and take it as safely and effectively as possible.

Five Reasons to Keep Herbal Antibiotics in Your Medicine Cabinet

We all know that feeling when we start to get sick – the scratchy throat, the sniffles, the fatigue. We also know the drill: head to the doctor for a prescription, fill it at the pharmacy and start popping pills.

But What If There Was a Better Way?

Herbal antibiotics are becoming increasingly popular as people look for alternatives to traditional medicine. There are plenty of good reasons to keep them in your medicine cabinet.

Effective

Herbal antibiotics have been used for centuries worldwide to treat everything from the common cold to more serious bacterial infections. They can also be as effective as traditional antibiotics.

Natural and Safe

Herbal antibiotics are made from natural ingredients like plants and herbs. They're generally much gentler on your body than synthetic drugs and have fewer side effects.

Boost Your Immune System

Another benefit of herbal antibiotics is that they help to boost your immune system. That's important because a robust immune system is your best defense against getting sick in the first place.

Inexpensive and Easy to Find

Herbal antibiotics are also usually much cheaper than traditional drugs. They're easy to find – often in your local health food store or online.

Good for the Environment

Traditional antibiotics are made from synthetic chemicals that can harm the environment. In contrast, herbal antibiotics are entirely natural and biodegradable.

How Are Herbal Antibiotics Different from Normal Antibiotics?

Herbal antibiotics work differently than traditional antibiotics. They are derived from natural sources, making them more effective in targeting infection. Herbal antibiotics have many bactericidal, bacteriostatic, and disinfectant activities and are an alternative against bacterial infections.

Additionally, herbal antibiotics often have fewer side effects because they are not as harsh on the body. Also, they don't kill good bacteria with the bad. Herbal antibiotics are generally non-toxic and ideal for treating bacterial infections in patients with a weakened immune system.

Pharmaceutical companies are interested in herbal antibiotics because they offer a potential new class. Herbal antibiotics are effective against many bacteria but are not always effective against all strains of a particular bacteria. The efficacy of herbal antibiotics can vary depending on the infection stage, the illness's severity, and the individual's response to treatment.

Are There Any Side Effects?

The side effects of herbal antibiotics depend on each specific plant and the dosage administered. In general, herbal antibiotics have fewer side effects than synthetic antibiotics.

Herbal antibiotics are generally non-toxic and much lower than synthetic antibiotics. In addition, they have fewer side effects and drug interactions than synthetic antibiotics. Reports of allergic reactions to herbal antibiotics are generally rare.

So, before you reach for those antibiotics, try herbal alternatives; they might do the trick. If all else fails, talk to your doctor about your best option. Antibiotics are a powerful tool for fighting infection, but they're not always necessary. With so many natural alternatives available, there's no need to resort to harsh chemicals when Mother Nature has already provided us with everything we need.

Chapter 3

Systemic Herbal Antibiotics

Systemic antibiotics are antibiotics taken orally and treat microbial infections of various types in the body. Antibiotics produced by microorganisms have been used for centuries to inhibit microbes' growth or to kill infectious microorganisms. With the discovery of more antibiotic-containing herbs and roots, it has become a common practice to include these herbal antibiotics in meals as regular ingredients for systemic function. When you regularly include herbal antibiotics in your diet, it helps prevent inflammation and microbial infection, promoting overall health. Although the health benefits of these herbs and ingredients are overwhelming, you should be careful not to overdo them to avoid causing harm to your body.

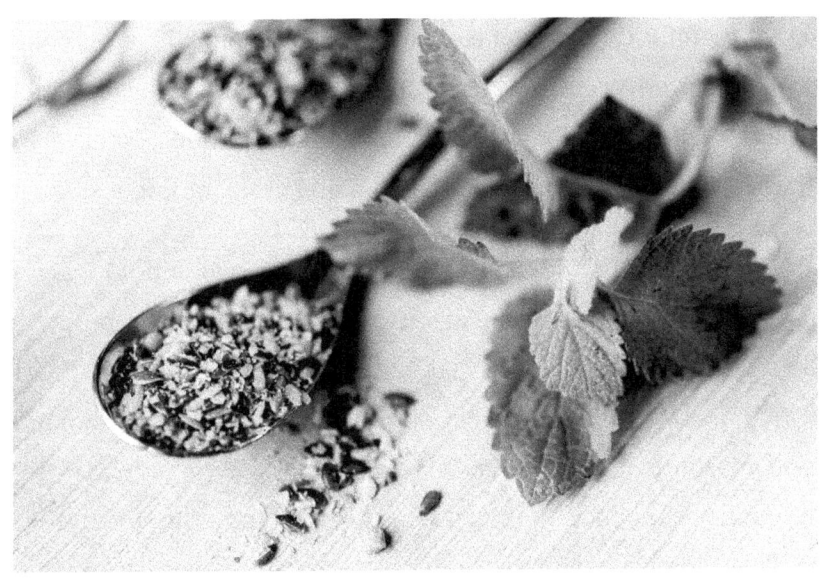

Common Use of Systemic Herbal Antibiotic

Systemic herbal antibiotics are commonly used when an infection has not occurred or is detected. It's taken to prevent the spread of diseases that, if unchecked, could prove fatal or severe. Herbal antibiotics are used to speed up recovery from injury or illness and to prevent further complications. People prone to microbial infection due to compromised health use these antibiotics regularly to avoid complications.

Ailments Treated with Herbal Antibiotics

Over the years, people have been turning to herbal antibiotics instead of chemically infused ones. Organic ingredients don't take a toll on the body as pharmaceutical medicines do. Antibiotics can exhaust the digestive system, whereas natural antibiotics are smoothly processed and digested.

Herbal antibiotics can treat or at least provide some level of control for a wide variety of illnesses. Inflammation, bacterial infections, urinary tract infections, diarrhea, wound injuries, and fungal infections can be treated or managed with herbal antibiotics.

The herbs and ingredients listed below are natural antibiotics. Each has unique properties allowing it to exhibit antibiotic properties. Oregano, Clove, Goldenseal, Echinacea, Ginger, Honey, Garlic, Neem, Pau D'Arco, Turmeric, Cabbage, Coconut Oil, and Fermented Food are some of these herbs. All these herbs and ingredients will be thoroughly explained to reveal their role in promoting overall well-being.

Oregano

Oregano is an herb used in many cuisines and supermarkets around the world. You can find it in oil, dried, or fresh form; no matter how you use it, it contains important health benefits. Oregano is consumed in small amounts, but because of its rich nutrient content, it will provide you with daily health benefits like vitamin K and aids in the fight against bacteria, resulting in less inflammation. This herb is high in antioxidants, helping the body fight free radicals, which are harmful to the body. When these free radicals are not removed and accumulate, they cause heart disease and cancer.

Thymol and carvacrol are antioxidants found in oregano oil that help prevent cell damage caused by free radicals. The antioxidant property also aids in preventing cancer. In addition to cancer prevention, professionals have claimed that oregano kills cancer cells. Compounds in essential oil have active antimicrobial properties. According to research, oregano inhibits the growth of microorganisms that cause infection, like pseudomonas and Escherichia coli. Certain viruses are also protected against by oregano components. Thymol and carvacrol are two powerful antiviral and antimicrobial components of oregano. Carvacrol deactivates norovirus, which causes diarrhea, stomach pain, and nausea. Oregano essential oil is proven to deactivate 90% of the herpes virus.

This herb is easy to incorporate into your diet, and its exceptional properties make it ideal as an antibiotic to combat viral infection, free radical complication, bacterial infection, and inflammation. Oregano is a natural food you can add to almost all your meals. However, a teaspoon amount is sufficient for your daily needs to avoid abusing the substance.

Clove

Cloves are the flower buds of the clove tree. It is available in grocery stores on the ground and in the whole form. Cloves are used as a seasoning, a spice in cakes and cookies, or a flavoring in hot beverages. Since cloves can be used in different dishes, it might lead you to believe that people only enjoy them for their flavor and aroma. However, this ingredient offers so much more. Clove has many health benefits, including blood sugar stabilization and liver health promotion. A teaspoon of clove powder contains enough minerals, vitamins, and antioxidants to help reduce oxidative stress.

Eugenol is a compound in clove that acts as a natural antioxidant, making it useful in the fight against oxidative stress. This means that clove can help protect against cancer. When clove is taken regularly, it inhibits tumor growth and kills cancer cells. However, don't consume large amounts of eugenol to avoid causing harm to your body.

Clove contains antibacterial properties, making it a natural antibiotic. Clove essential oil is highly potent and protects you from food poisoning. Clove also promotes oral health by preventing bacteria growth that causes gum disease; regularly brushing your teeth with a clove paste will strengthen gum health. Clove is classified as an herbal antibiotic due to its antimicrobial properties.

Onion

Onion belongs to the Allium genius family and is one of the vegetables high in minerals, vitamins, and other health benefits. Since ancient times, the medicinal benefits of onion have been used to treat many ailments such as heart disease, mouth sores, and headaches. One of the many remarkable properties of onion is vitamin C, an antioxidant in the body; this antioxidant shields the body from free radicals. The antibiotic property stems from onion's ability to fight inflammation and bacteria, but it also has various other medicinal properties. It prevents blood clots and high blood pressure. Additionally, Onion extract inhibits the growth of Vibrio cholerae, the bacteria responsible for cholera infection.

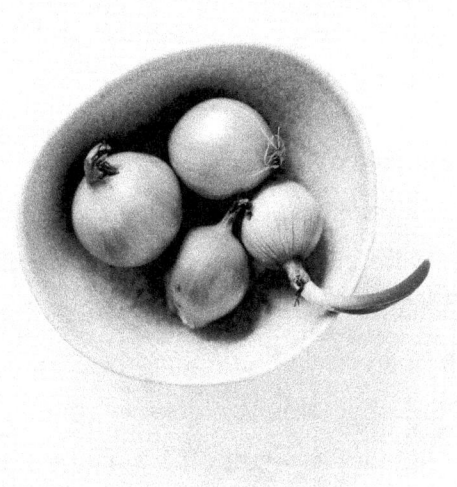

Several bacteria, including E. coli and S. aureus, that cause various diseases in the gastrointestinal tract and stomach, have been rendered inactive by the inhibitory action of onions, particularly red onions. This vegetable is readily available in grocery stores worldwide, and you can incorporate it into all your meals to reap the benefits. Aside from the bulb, the onion leaves are edible and high in nutrients that promote overall health.

Goldenseal

This herb is native to North America and is known as yellow puccoon or orangeroot. Its dried root is widely used as a supplement in the United States. Berberine is a goldenseal component that aids in the fight against fungi and bacteria infection. Aside from its antimicrobial properties, it reduces irregular heartbeat and blood pressure. Goldenseal can treat colds, hay fever, upper respiratory tract infections, constipation, and diarrhea. Although there is no medical basis for these treatments, they have been performed and confirmed through research. The leaves and roots of goldenseal treat conditions like inflammation and infection.

Goldenseal is a well-known herbal medicine used all over the world. Its herbal extracts and teas treat hay fever, colds, digestive issues, skin issues, and sore gums. It is also processed and used in many medications, including allergy relief products, ear drops, feminine hygiene products, eyewash formulations, laxatives, flu and cold remedies, and digestive aids. Goldenseal contains a high alkaloid concentration, giving it anti-inflammatory and antibacterial properties, making it an herbal antibiotic. Aside from its antibiotic properties, goldenseal can help with appetite loss, skin disorders, painful or heavy periods, indigestion, sinus infection, and other digestive or inflammatory disorders.

Honey

Honey is made by bees using nectar from flowers. Honey is a sweet liquid used medicinally for centuries due to its many purported health benefits. You can purchase raw honey or pasteurized honey. The pasteurization process results in a darker or lighter shade of honey. The sweetness of honey comes from its high glucose content and has successfully been used to treat seasonal allergies. But it can do so much more for your body. Honey also aids in the speedy recovery of burns and other wounds when applied topically. Other body products like shampoo, deodorant, and creams contain honey in different quantities because of its health benefit. People with diabetes cannot benefit from honey because they risk sugar breakdown.

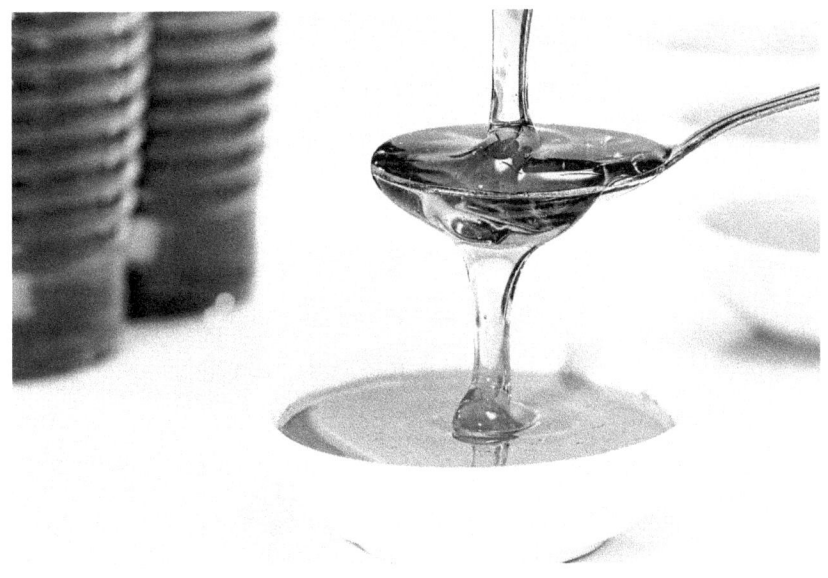

Because of its ability to fight infection and inhibit microbial growth, honey is regarded as a natural antibiotic. Although other honey types have antibacterial properties, professionals found that Manuka honey has a higher antibacterial ability. Manuka honey contains defensen-1 proteins and hydrogen peroxide, which aid in killing bacteria.

Honey can cure various ailments when taken alone or combined with other solutions, including bad breath, teething pain, dermatitis and eczema, wounds, cuts, burns, asthma and cough, stomach ulcer, and arthritis. Due to its antioxidant, anti-inflammatory, anti-viral, and antibacterial properties, honey is recommended to treat many skin ailments. These properties qualify it as a natural antibiotic. Honey is easily available in grocery stores and in place of sugar in recipes. Even though honey has numerous health benefits, consuming too much can harm your health.

Echinacea

Coneflowers are the common name for the various Echinacea species and are easily found throughout North America's middle and eastern parts. This plant's medicinal properties come from roots, flowers, and leaves.

Consuming echinacea stimulates the production of a chemical within the body that reduces inflammation and strengthens the immune system. Echinacea is known for its anti-inflammatory and immune-enhancing properties and helps prevent the common cold in older people when taken orally regularly. Taking Echinacea when you already have a cold makes the supplement less effective than when you are in good health. Echinacea is included in skin care products because it aids in preventing skin infections. Echinacea's ability to reduce inflammation makes it a naturally occurring antibiotic easily integrated into culinary preparations.

Ginger

Ginger is derived from a flowering plant, and its rhizome is used as a spice in many cuisines due to its spicy nature and strong aroma. This flowering plant is indigenous to Southeast Asia and regarded as one of the world's healthiest spices. The underground stem, the rhizome, is most frequently used to season food.

Ginger can be utilized in dried, fresh, juiced, oil-infused, and powdered forms. It has a long history of medicinal use, including reducing nausea, improving digestion, and treating the common cold and flu. Gingerol is the bioactive component responsible for its medicinal properties. Additionally, it possesses antioxidant and anti-inflammatory properties. Ginger also aids in managing oxidative stress caused by an excess of free radicals in the body. Individuals suffering from nausea and vomiting due to medical conditions like chemotherapy or surgery can benefit from ginger.

Ginger can reduce nausea in pregnant women with morning sickness, but it cannot stop vomiting. It has been employed as an alternative medicine for decades due to its anti-cancer properties. This anti-cancer property is due to gingerol, abundant in raw ginger. Ginger can be effective against ovarian, breast, liver, and pancreatic cancers. It inhibits disease-causing bacteria's growth, so including it in your diet reduces your risk of bacterial infection. Ginger inhibits oral bacteria responsible for inflammatory gum infections such as periodontitis and gingivitis. Combating these dangerous viruses and bacteria reduces your likelihood of contracting an infection. Ginger is easily incorporated into your diet by drinking and eating. It is a natural antibiotic and has numerous health benefits, including antibiotic properties. Include ginger in your diet regularly to boost your immune system and fight infections.

Garlic

Garlic has numerous health benefits, including lowering cholesterol and blood pressure and preventing the common cold. It is remarkable how easily this ingredient can be incorporated into regular meals, protecting the body and sating the appetite. Garlic is an onion (allium) family member and origins in Northern Asia. It is easy to cultivate in many parts of the world, available in any supermarket, and its delicious flavor and pungent odor make it an excellent cooking ingredient.

Historically, garlic was primarily utilized for its medicinal and health benefits. When garlic is chewed, crushed, or chopped, a sulfur compound is released; this is responsible for its health benefits. This sulfur compound spreads systemically throughout the body and has a profound biological effect. Garlic can strengthen your immune system and help you combat the flu and the common cold. Garlic also contains antioxidants that aid in the prevention of Alzheimer's disease and dementia. Garlic is also effective against diarrhea, vomiting, and fungi.

Free radical-induced oxidative stress can accelerate aging, but garlic's antioxidants can prevent this from happening. As a natural antibiotic, garlic inhibits microbial infection. Include it in your diet to benefit from its systemic effect.

Pau D'Arco

This evergreen tree originated in South America and has been used for centuries due to its medicinal properties. The name derives from Portugal and means "bow tree." It is used in cancer and antibacterial treatment; the administration of the bow tree has been observed to slow tumor growth. According to research, it helps weight loss and reduces inflammation.

Bow tree is a natural antibiotic due to its ability to treat infections. Aside from the benefits already mentioned, the medicinal properties of the bow tree are enormous, and this herb helps with skin and stomach ailments. It is not recommended to consume in large quantities to avoid complications. People with bleeding issues or about to undergo surgery should avoid this herb because it slows blood clotting. The main components of Pau D' Arco that allow it to treat various illnesses are beta-lapachone and lapachol, classified as naphthoquinone.

The extract from pau d'arco has antifungal and antibacterial properties that inhibit fungi and bacteria metabolism, starving them to death. It employs an inhibition mechanism to keep your body safe from infection. It is best to consume in moderation to avoid the risk of overdosing.

Neem

Although it grows in other parts of the world, the neem tree originated in India. Neem oil treats bacterial skin infections like acne and dermatitis. This ingredient is a natural systemic antibiotic that should be consumed in moderation. Throughout history, the neem tree has been used to treat fever, pain, and infection, and its twigs are used to clean teeth, promoting dental care.

Neem is sometimes referred to as "the village pharmacy" because all parts of this medicinal plant, including the flowers, leaves, bark, roots, fruits, and seeds, are useful in treating various ailments. The flowers treat bile duct issues, the leaves treat ulcers, and the bark treats brain illnesses. More than 140 active compounds have been discovered in various parts of the neem tree. These powerful compounds have given neem its antimicrobial, antiparasitic, anti-inflammatory, wound-healing, antioxidant, and antidiabetic properties. The name 'village pharmacy' is well-deserved because this herb is extremely potent. Due to its ability to combat multiple infections, it is a natural antibiotic easily added to the diet for systemic results.

Turmeric

Turmeric acts as a soldier for the body. As a nutritional supplement, turmeric has the highest disease-fighting efficacy of all food ingredients. The health benefits of turmeric are due to curcumin, the active ingredient. The Indian herb and spice have been used medicinally for centuries. Curcumin, the active component of turmeric, possesses powerful anti-inflammatory and antioxidant properties.

Since raw turmeric contains only a small amount of curcumin, individuals take supplements to increase their curcumin intake. Poor absorption of curcumin into the bloodstream is a challenge that must be overcome by increasing the bioavailability of curcumin. Piperine, present in black pepper, enhances the absorption and efficacy of curcumin by 2,000%. For optimal results, it is recommended to combine turmeric and black pepper. Curcumin is anti-inflammatory and aids the body's defense against foreign invaders while repairing internal damage. Only by increasing its bioavailability can curcumin inhibit molecules crucial in inflammation.

Turmeric increases your body's antioxidant capacity and lengthens your lifespan. Its ability to prevent or treat infections caused by microorganisms makes turmeric a highly sought-after natural antibiotic. It combats microorganisms causing infections and is easily incorporated into the diet.

Cabbage

Cabbage, belonging to the cruciferous family, contains a high sulfur content. It comes in different colors, including green, white, purple, and red, and its leaves can be smooth or crinkled. Cabbage is grown worldwide and included in various dishes, such as coleslaw, kimchi, and sauerkraut. It is available in any vegetable store or supermarket.

Cabbage uses its antioxidant properties to help prevent inflammation caused by infection or disease. It contains vitamin C, which is important for many bodily functions, and aids in forming collagen, which gives your skin flexibility and structure. Collagen is essential for properly functioning blood vessels, muscles, and bones. This food aids in the fight against cancer and improves weight management, digestion issues, and disease prevention. Cabbage is natural and can be included in various diets to reap its antibiotic properties and benefits.

Fermented Food

Pickles, probiotic yogurt, and unpasteurized cabbage are some examples of fermented foods beneficial to health. It contributes to the fight against cancer and bacterial infection. The acidic content of raw food can be reduced through fermentation, ultimately resulting in healthier food. Fermented food has been made for many years in different cultures all over the world. Fermented foods are beneficial to the body because they enhance immunity, reduce the risk of allergic reactions, eliminate harmful microbes and yeast, and provide numerous health benefits. Typically, fermented foods are considered natural antibiotics because they help fight microbial infections - for example, vinegar made from apple cider.

The antiseptic and antibiotic properties this vinegar possesses make it ideal for treating and preventing infections. In addition, it helps reduce the risk of cancer and cholesterol. When apple cider is applied to wounds, it shields the body from infections that could develop due to contamination that the wound might have been exposed to. This natural remedy has a long history of application in the kitchen and the medical field. Using apple cider vinegar has several positive effects on health, including lowering cholesterol and blood sugar levels and making it easier to shed excess weight.

This treatment is made from fermented apple sugar, and as a result of the fermentation process, the apple sugar molecules transform into acetic acid. The acetic acid present in this treatment is the component responsible for the positive health effects associated with apple cider vinegar. Since it acts as a natural antibiotic, you should make it a regular part of your diet for the most benefit.

Nature offers a wide range of nutritious foods. Its functionality is systemic because it has no specific organ or cell to work on. Interestingly, almost every natural food we eat has one or more health benefits. These natural antibiotics discussed in this chapter are taken orally and circulate throughout the body, performing their functions. Most of these herbs and ingredients work best when consumed before illness rather than when the illness is fully activated; they prevent disease by inhibiting the disease-causing organism. Making it a regular part of your diet will go a long way toward keeping your body healthy.

Chapter 4

Non-Systemic Herbal Antibiotics

Herbal antibiotics, among other medications, have been used for a long time as treatments for various illnesses by healers and herbalists. In recent years, these natural remedies have gained even more prominence from the public.

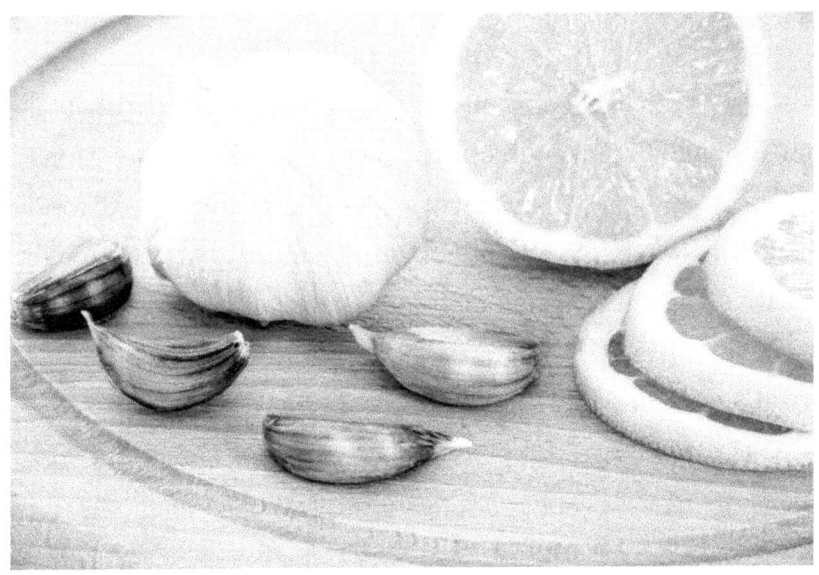

Since the synthetic drugs that helped build modern medicine are failing, herbal medicine is once again getting the attention it deserves. Herbal antibiotics have a good chance of becoming a standard treatment option.

Since 1928, when antibiotics were discovered, bacteria have changed and adapted faster than anyone could have imagined. So, the need for safer and more effective treatments is more urgent than ever. It has led many professionals and ordinary people to look to nature and the healing powers of the earth once again. Therefore, many plants and herbs our ancestors once used are again being sought.

In the further search for new treatments against antibiotic-resistant organisms, numerous plants and herbs with antibacterial properties have been discovered. Like their synthetic counterparts, these herbal antibiotics can be broken down into two categories: systemic and non-systemic.

With the rise in deadly infections, it is important to know about these non-systemic herbal antibiotics—where they can be found, and the various types. This chapter covers everything you need to know about non-systemic herbal antibiotics, their use, where to find them, and what ailments they are used for.

What Are Non-Systemic Antibiotics?

Non-systemic antibiotics, known as localized antibiotics, do not spread across the body as easily as systemic antibiotics; their movements are limited because they cannot easily cross through membranes. These antibiotics are only active in the gastrointestinal and urinary tract. In external infections, they only act in the intestinal lumen without reaching the systemic circulation areas. Even though they only work on the digestive system, they can treat more than just GI infections.

Non-systemic antibiotics can treat various systemic diseases, including metabolic and mineral imbalances.

Non-systemic antibiotics provide a much-needed solution in a world where safety is vital. It is about using herbal antibiotics and the approval process for large-scale ailment medications, those treating chronic diseases affecting a large patient population.

These antibiotics help reduce and, in some cases, eliminate off-target systemic effects, reducing toxic and adverse effect risks. Non-systemic antibiotics have good therapeutic potential because they can address unfulfilled medical needs by providing innovative treatment options with minimal adverse effects.

Ailments Assisted by Non-Systemic Antibiotics

Non-systemic antibiotics treat a wide range of infections in the body, especially bacterial infections in the digestive tract. This antibacterial has a high bactericidal activity, making it effective against bacteria, aerobes, and anaerobes. Here are some examples of illnesses that can be treated with non-systemic antibiotics:

Hepatic Encephalopathy

This disease is a loss of brain function caused by a damaged liver's inability to remove toxins in the blood. It commonly occurs in people with chronic liver disease and is usually triggered by dehydration, gastrointestinal bleeding, or infection.

Early symptoms include mild forgetfulness, excessive sleepiness, a misty sweet odor on the breath, and confusion. Advanced symptoms include flapping tremors (trembling of the hands and arms), stirred speech, disorientation, and coma.

Hepatic encephalopathy can be treated in various ways, including using non-systemic antibiotics to inhibit and kill the bacteria. Using non-systemic antibiotics works quickly, reducing the possibility of hospitalization.

Inflammatory Bowel Disease

Inflammatory Bowel Disease, known as IBD, is divided into two types: ulcerative colitis and Crohn's disease. These disorders are characterized by a long history of chronic tissue inflammation within the digestive tract, affecting the small and large intestines, colon, rectum, and upper gastrointestinal tract.

The severity of this disease varies depending on the individual infected. It can be a minor infection in one person or a life-threatening condition in another. This disease is distinguished by symptoms such as rectal bleeding, fatigue, diarrhea, weight loss, and abdominal pain.

This disease can be treated with non-systemic antibiotics and several other medications to kill the bacteria.

Cholera

Cholera is a common bacterial infection. It is an acute infection caused by bacterial contamination of food or drink, causing watery diarrhea and dehydration.

In extreme situations, severe dehydration and diarrhea could be accompanied by shock and seizures. It can lead to death in a matter of days or even hours if not treated quickly. Localized or non-systemic antibacterial can treat cholera effectively.

Small Intestinal Bacteria Overgrowth (SIBO)

Small intestinal bacteria overgrowth happens when the increase in bacteria inside the small intestine is abnormal. It is a result of bacteria not being native to the digestive tract region. This illness is caused by disease or surgery, which disturbs the movement of waste products and food through the digestive system, creating a space for bacteria to thrive. They contribute to structural issues within the body.

This disease is associated with nausea, diarrhea, weight loss, bloating, loss of appetite, abdominal pain, and other symptoms. Antibiotics are used to kill and remove overgrown bacteria. Non-systemic antibiotics reduce the abnormal bacteria growing in the digestive tract. The duration of this treatment depends solely on the patient.

Infected Wounds

Bacteria are the most common microbes that infect wounds. These bacteria and other microbes get into the wound and use it as a place to grow, making the wound take longer to heal. An example of these bacteria is staphylococcus aureus.

Wounds already infected become even more infected, and areas of the wound that appear red will feel slightly warm or hot. The wound becomes more painful and might produce pus, a smelly yellowish liquid.

Non-systemic antibiotics are excellent for treating wounds infected by bacteria. These bacteria can't grow where an antibacterial is applied so the wound can heal properly.

Herbs and Ingredients Used as Natural Antibiotics

Researchers and scientists are turning to natural methods to develop new drugs because bacteria quickly change and adapt to synthetic drugs, making them less effective.

Using natural remedies such as antibiotics instead of well-known synthetic drugs has several advantages. These benefits are less chance of side effects, general availability, better effectiveness in long-term cases, and lower cost.

Below is a list of the most effective natural antibiotics that can be used as an alternative to synthetic drugs. These natural antibiotics have the potential to become a standard treatment method.

Garlic

Garlic, botanically known as Allium sativum, is a perennial plant in the amaryllis family (Amaryllidaceae). It is shaped like a bulb, covered with a membrane skin and smaller bulblets known as cloves enclosed within it.

This plant is native to central Asia, but it is now widely grown in Italy and parts of southern France.

Garlic is widely used as a staple ingredient in various cuisines around the world due to its pungent flavor and aroma. Besides its delicious flavor, garlic has long been used as medicine for many ailments in ancient and modern times. One of its many health and therapeutic benefits is its antibiotic properties.

Garlic cloves treat bacterial infections of the skin, digestive tract, respiratory tract, and urinary tract. Bacteria cannot adapt to garlic because it is composed of multiple components rather than a single compound. Garlic contains 33 sulfur compounds, 17 amino acids, and many more.

Antibiotic Properties

Because of its active sulfur component, allicin, garlic is considered a natural antibiotic. When treating an infection in the gut caused by Campylobacter bacteria, this compound is a hundred times stronger and more effective than some popular antibiotics.

Juniper

Junipers are members of the Cupressaceae family and the genus Juniperus. Their trees and shrubs are coniferous and grow in western, southern, and central Asia, southern and tropical Africa, the Arctic, eastern Tibet, and Central American mountains.

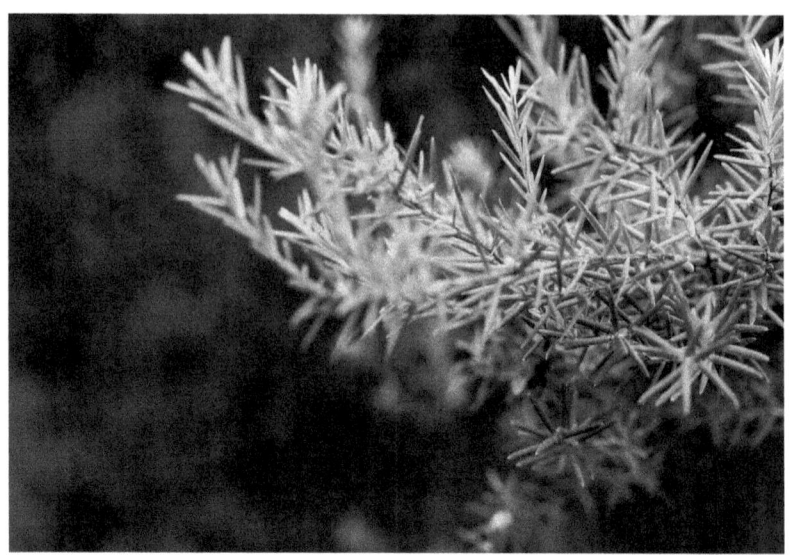

Junipers come in various shapes and sizes, ranging from tall trees to low shrubs, with trailing long branches and needle-like leaves. Its fruits are shaped like berries and are blue, orange, or reddish brown.

Juniper berries are aromatic and commonly used as a spice in cooking. The berries and needle-like leaves are commonly used for herbal purposes. The roots and bark of the tree are also active.

Juniper berries have antiseptic properties and treat chronic urinary tract infections. It accomplishes healing by facilitating urinary passages, allowing for faster fluid movement in the kidneys. Juniper is extremely beneficial in renal insufficiency (when the kidney works slowly) and restricted urine flow. It is used to treat skin infections by removing toxins from the blood.

Also, it treats eczema, acne, and other skin infections like dandruff and athlete's foot. Proceed with caution and under the supervision of a medical expert when using juniper.

Antibiotic Properties

Juniper oil contains powerful and effective compounds, such as sabinene, myrcene, limonene, and alpha and beta-pinene. It also contains thujene and terpene, which form an antiseptic barrier and are beneficial in treating kidney diseases, digestive disorders, and enlarged prostate. It is also high in vitamin C.

Honey

Honey is a viscous liquid with a dark golden color produced by bees in their honey sacs. The flower from the nectar determines the color and flavor of the honey. It can be purchased raw or pasteurized.

Honey has numerous applications. When applied as a protective coating, it is a soothing component on the skin and heals wounds, burns, sores, and skin grafts. Honey treats the common cold, asthma, phlegm, and cough. It also stabilizes the liver, relieves pain, and eliminates toxins.

Antibiotic Properties

Honey has a high viscosity and contains an antibacterial enzyme that produces hydrogen peroxide, which inhibits bacteria growth. It is useful in treating stomach ulcers and the bacterium Helicobacter pylori.

Echinacea

The genus name Echinacea refers to a group of flowering plants in the daisy family. This plant is native to North America and is known as coneflower. Its flowers are purple or pink, depending on the species. The petals surrounding the cone are spiky and red or dark brown.

This plant is related to ragweed and sunflowers; the leaves, roots, and flowers are used medicinally to reduce inflammation and boost the immune system. It is a well-known natural remedy used to boost immunity by producing active germ-fighting cells in our bodies. It also treats the common cold and flu.

Echinacea is known to inhibit bacteria by preventing them from releasing an enzyme known as hyaluronidase, allowing bacteria to break through protective membranes such as the lining of the respiratory and intestinal tracts and invading tissues. It also prevents some viruses, like flu viruses.

Antibiotic Properties

Polysaccharides, alkamides, flavonoids, glycoproteins, and volatile oils are all found in Echinacea. It also has an immunostimulant, which helps the immune system fight upper respiratory tract infections by making them stronger.

Cranberry

This plant belongs to the genus Vaccinium and the subgenus Oxycoccus; they are short, evergreen shrubs or trailing vines in the

Ericaceae family. This plant is high in phytonutrients, particularly proanthocyanin antioxidants, and essential for overall health.

Cranberries also aid in preventing oral diseases such as caries and gingivitis by preventing food particles and bacteria from sticking to your teeth. They also contain components that protect against illnesses like urinary tract infections, tooth decay, and other inflammatory diseases.

Antibiotic Properties

Cranberry is primarily used to treat urinary tract infections. It contains proanthocyanins, flavonoids, and phenolic acid, which work together to form a protective barrier around the urinary tract.

Licorice Root

Licorice root is an herb used in herbal medicine for many years to treat ailments such as stomach aches, coughs, infections, asthma, insomnia, inflammation, upper respiratory tract issues, and soothing digestive tract problems.

It is also used as a sweetener in beverages, medicine, and candies. Licorice has numerous health benefits, including antioxidants, anti-inflammatory, and antimicrobial properties.

Licorice root is grown in Europe, Asia, and some parts of the Middle East.

It also contains antidepressant compounds. These compounds allow it to treat athletes' foot, bursitis, cold and flu, emphysema, heartburn, tuberculosis, ulcers, fungal infections, yeast infections, tooth decay, canker sores, arthritis, psoriasis, liver disease, gingivitis, fatigue, sore throat, gout, and many other conditions.

Antibiotic properties

Glycyrrhizin is found in licorice roots; this aids in healing the mucous membranes in the digestive tract, thereby healing the gastrointestinal system. Licorice roots also treat stomach inflammation.

Olive Leaf

Olives are plants that belong to the Oleaceae family. Its botanical name is Olea europaea, and it belongs to the drapes or stone family of fruits. This fruit is consumed or extracted for its oil.

Olives contain a high concentration of plant compounds known as polyphenols, which have antioxidant and anti-inflammatory properties. Polyphenols help lower blood pressure and bad cholesterol while preventing cancer. It also helps protect against oxidative damage and cognitive decline. Anti-inflammatory and antioxidant properties potentially treat atherosclerosis, cancer, arthritis, neurodegenerative diseases, and diabetes.

It has also been linked to preventing snoring and lowering cholesterol levels.

Antibiotic Properties

Oleuropein is a unique molecule found in olives. It is primarily used to lower blood pressure and cholesterol by breaking down the walls of pathogenic bacteria cells.

Eucalyptus

Eucalyptus oil is one of the purest essential oils. The oil is made from the eucalyptus globulus tree, also called "blue gum," and is available globally. It is native to Australia and is an evergreen tree with a rapid growth rate.

Since it is extracted from dried eucalyptus leaves, the oil has numerous healing properties. It aids in treating asthma, bronchitis, malaria, whopping cough, oral health problems, gallbladder problems, and other ailments.

Antibiotic Properties

Eucalyptus contains volatile oil and flavonoids, which kill bacteria, and provides respiratory relief for blocked noses, sinusitis, and coughs.

Ginseng

Ginseng is the root of plants in the genus Panax. They are grown in South China, America, and Korea. Ginseng is typically characterized by its gametocides and gintonin. Although other herbs exist and are called ginseng, they lack the active ingredient ginsenosides.

Ginseng is used to prevent premature aging. It also helps improve mental health and cognitive power, energizing the body and reducing tiredness.

Antibodies Properties

The active component in ginseng is ginsenosides, which help in many areas of the body by increasing resistance to stress and vitality. It also treats respiratory tract infections, diabetes, and debility.

Shatavari

Shatavari, known as asparagus racemous, is a climbing plant native to India's low jungles. This herb tastes both sweet and bitter. It is considered the complete opposite of Ashwagandha in India. It has rejuvenating effects on the reproductive organs of females. Shatavari can treat various ailments in men and women, such as rheumatism, headaches, diarrhea, coughing, and alcohol withdrawal. Shatavari is a remedy found in most herbal stores.

Antibiotic Properties

Shatavari contains arurveda, which boosts antibacterial activity in the body, making it an excellent herb for preventing and fighting bacterial infections. It also treats digestive problems and oophorectomy, and hysterectomy recovery.

Shitake Mushrooms

Shitake mushrooms are known in Asia to represent longevity due to their numerous health-enhancing properties. The Chinese have used this mushroom medicinally for over 6,000 years. Aside from its various health benefits, such as asthma, flu, bronchitis, anti-aging, tumors, and cancer, the shitake mushroom is also an amazing ingredient in specialty cuisines.

The mushroom's delicious taste in food led to its adoption across the United States and the rest of the world. It can be found in food and health stores near you. Depending on your needs, it can be consumed in food, as a capsule, powder, or extract.

Antibiotic Properties

The shitake mushroom contains Lenticular edodes, which can kill many bacterial pathogens. It is used to maintain and protect the immune system.

Goldenseal

The North American goldenseal, known as orangeroot, is a perennial plant in the buttercup family, Ranunculaceae. It is identifiable by its thick, golden, tangled rootstock. Above ground, the stem is purple and hairy, while below ground, it becomes yellow at the point where it joins the rhizome.

In the United States, dried roots are widely utilized in nutritional supplements.

Goldenseal has antibacterial and antifungal properties. It has blood pressure-lowering qualities and helps with irregular heartbeats. However, most of the essential compounds in goldenseal are poorly absorbed when taken orally.

Goldenseal treats many health problems, such as colds, respiratory infections, constipation, diarrhea, and fever.

Antibiotic Properties

Berberine, a chemical in goldenseal, has been shown in laboratory trials to kill some bacteria and fungi. However, goldenseal's antibacterial properties have led to treating many conditions, including ocular infections, gastrointestinal infections, urinary infections, mouth sores, and even vaginitis.

Oregano

Oregano, known as Marjoram, is a member of the Lamiaceae family. It is a plant native to the Mediterranean and is common in parts of North America. It is a perennial used as a spice in cooking and making medicinal herbs.

It has dark oval leaves and fragrant spike-shaped flowers in purple, pink, or white. Although it is widely used as a spice in cooking and as a fragrance component in scented oils, perfumes, cosmetics, detergents, etc., many people are unaware of its amazing antibiotic properties. It can be purchased in health food stores and herbal remedy shops.

Herbalists frequently use oregano as a preservative or as an antidote against poison. The oil obtained from its leaves and flowers greatly protects against infections caused by harmful bacteria. It also treats menstrual cramps by chewing on about 4 to 5 of its freshly cut leaves. Besides menstrual cramps, oregano is excellent anti-aging food. Additionally, oregano can treat other conditions such as asthma, influenza, cuts and bruises, acne, dandruff, muscle pain, varicose veins, wrinkles, etc.

Antibiotic Properties

Carvacrol and thymol are natural compounds in oregano. These compounds aid in the breakdown of the bacterium's outer cell membrane, a barrier between the bacteria and our body's immune system. Therefore, oregano aids in the death of bacteria. As a result, it is primarily used to treat candidiasis and respiratory tract infections.

Uva-ursi

Arctostaphylos Uva-ursi, known as Uva-ursi, is an evergreen shrub in the Ericaceae family. Its English name is Bearberry, and it grows in the northern regions of North America in sandy and rocky woods and open areas in Asia and Europe. This flowering shrub grows about 30 centimeters in height, with trailing stems and flowers and leaves clustering at the tips of the branches. It also produces a reddish-orange berry that bears enjoy, hence, its name.

Bearberry leaves have a slight aroma and an extremely bitter taste when dried. The leaves are occasionally boiled and drunk as tea. The fruit's bland flavor improves when cooked. Aside from being used as an edible, Uva-ursi has numerous medicinal benefits. It is a laxative to prevent constipation and aid digestion and is primarily used to treat urinary tract infections. Additionally, it treats cystitis, urethritis, bronchitis, bloating, kidney and bladder infections, and other conditions.

Antibiotic Properties

Ellagic, gallic acid tannins, and hydrolyzable are some of the antibiotic properties in Uva-ursi. Arbutin is the primary bioactive responsible for its antibacterial properties. When arbutin is released through urine, it produces a metabolite called Hydroquinone glucuronide, which prevents bacteria from adhering to tissues in that area.

It is clear that non-systemic herbal antibiotics are safe and an excellent alternative to conventional and synthetic medicine. Natural remedies have several advantages over their synthetic counterparts, including fewer side effects, greater accessibility, lower costs, and greater efficiency. These antibiotics can be consumed in various ways, including food, herbs, oils, medicines, spices, and tablets. They assist you in fighting and protecting yourself against all harmful microbes.

Chapter 5

Synergist Antibiotics

There are major concerns for medical science in our constantly changing world. These concerns range from mutated pathogens to resilient parasites and resistant bacteria. Finding new ways to combat diseases and epidemics while improving people's lives requires a high level of expertise. Intensive study, research, and experiments are required to combat diseases in any form.

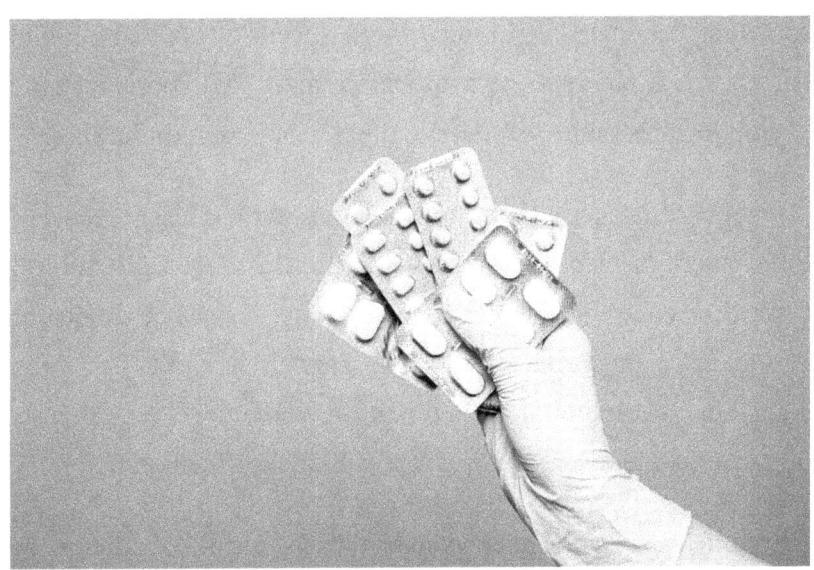

What Does 'Synergist Antibiotics' Mean?

Antibiotic synergism is among the novel ways of treating bacterial infections. Antibiotic synergy is a microbiological phenomenon occurring when two bioactive agents are combined for increased potency against bacteria. Antimicrobial drugs have a property known as synergism that makes them more effective when taken together. This phenomenon arose due to resistant bacteria and pathogens that refused to be treated with a single antibacterial medication.

Antibiotic synergy is defined as the response observed when two or more antibacterial antibiotics are used to treat an infection simultaneously. The combined antibiotics work together to produce a stronger effect or result than if the antibiotics were used individually. The antibiotics work better together than they do separately, so the bacteria or pathogen has less chance of surviving.

Following an increase in reports in recent years, antimicrobial resistance has emerged as a global concern. Microorganisms can develop mechanisms to neutralize the potency of antimicrobials.

Antibiotic resistance relates to synergist antibiotics, which is the development of mechanisms to withstand the effects of antibiotics, eventually rendering them ineffective. This resistance could result from genetic mutation, which can happen naturally or through acquisition from similar bacteria in the same species. Overuse of antibiotics could also influence reducing their effectiveness.

Antibiotic resistance occurs when bacteria's response to medications changes. This resistance develops in the bacteria infecting animals and humans, not in the good bacteria of animals and humans. Infections caused by antibiotic-resistant bacteria are more difficult to treat than infections caused by non-resistant strains. This resistance has greatly contributed to increased mortality, prolonged stays in hospitals and clinics, and increased medical costs, significantly threatening the quality and longevity of human and animal life.

Every year, medical conditions caused by this resistance result in a large number of deaths. Antibiotic resistance has made it harder and more expensive to treat infections. So, the idea of antibiotic synergy has come about.

Medical interest in synergist antibiotics dates back to the early 1950s. Doctors noticed a high relapse rate in patients with enterococcal endocarditis treated solely with penicillin G. However, there was a remarkably low relapse rate when penicillin G was combined with streptomycin to treat the infection. Since that discovery, the medical research community has been questioning and contemplating the possibilities and effects of antibiotic combinations.

Combination therapy is currently acknowledged as providing a broad spectrum of antibiotic protection, optimally fighting polymicrobial infections, reducing dose toxicity when necessary, limiting selections for antibiotic-resistant strains, and, in some cases, exhibiting synergistic activity.

Antibiotic combinations have been widely used in response to the rise in the number of reported cases of resistant strains of bacterial infections. This rapid spread of antibiotic-resistant diseases has prompted using antibiotic combinations to combat bacterial resistance and evolution while maintaining medical efficacy.

Antibiotics work together to produce inhibitory effects stronger than the individual potencies of each drug. There is an argument that synergist antibiotics cause side effects. However, they can be kept at desirable medically satisfactory levels if administered clinically.

Antibiotic synergy combats and defeats the infection quickly, reducing the time it takes for resistant strains to emerge. However, it increases the advantage of mutant strains over wild-type cells. If the combination is used correctly, it creates more synergy, which lowers the risk of bacteria resistant to more than one drug.

A few other reasons support using synergist antibiotics in treating bacterial infections. Some of these reasons are stated below.

- Broad spectrum therapy coverage for adversely affected patients
- Prevention of polymicrobial infections
- Preventing the possible selection of bacteria resistant to antibiotics where the microbe changes quickly in response to the drug.
- Lowering dose-related toxicity, which is unprecedented and historically significant.

When synergistic antibiotics are used together, they treat specific bacterial infections. Antibiotics' synergistic activity combats infections caused by resistant bacterial strains or infections requiring bacterial eradication. The combined antibiotics' increased potency treats these infections.

Common Use of Synergistic Antibiotics

Although bacterial resistance to medications is a major threat to human health, some infections can still be treated with a single medication. Synergist antibiotics are typically prescribed for bacterial strains that have developed resistance to a specific drug, rendering it ineffective. It is also given to people with a low immune system and whose bodies cannot produce antibodies that cooperate with the antibiotics or be stimulated by the antibiotics to fight the infection.

Antibiotic synergy is desirable for several additional reasons. Synergist antibiotics produce more antibacterial potency at the patient level, allowing the body to quickly rid itself of infections and resulting in less time spent on antibiotic therapy.

The primary purpose of using synergist antibiotics is to combat infection from antibacterial resistant strains and to prevent spreading bacterial resistance through infection eradication. Before they can be used therapeutically, these antibiotics are tested in vitro and in animal forms for clinical significance.

The availability and use of effective antibiotics are crucial in some fields of modern medicine. Without effective antibiotics, it would not be possible to do organ transplants, chemotherapy to treat cancer, intensive care for premature babies, hip replacement surgery, and other procedures.

These antibiotics can treat human and animal illnesses. They combat antibiotic-resistant strains in humans and animals. These resistant strains significantly threaten global health, food security, and food safety. They have developed resistance to common medicine to treat them. As a result, synergist antibiotics have provided a way to avert this crisis following extensive research by the pharmacological and medical communities.

Many bacteria strains have developed resistance to various antibiotics, including:

- Methicillin-Resistant Staphylococcus Aureus (MRSA).
- Bacteria strain responsible for multi-drug resistant tuberculosis.
- Clostridium difficile.
- Escherichia Coli
- Neisseria Gonorrhoeae.
- Vancomycin-Resistant Enterococcus (VRE)
- Enterobacteriaceae (gut bacteria)

Pneumonia, urinary and respiratory infections, intestinal diseases, and tuberculosis have become more difficult to treat, making single antibiotics less effective. Other antibiotic-resistant infections include blood poisoning, ear and chest infections, sore throats, foodborne diseases, and gonorrhea. This growing list has become a concern globally, and combining antibiotics to create a more potent approach to fighting them is now a popular option.

MRSA, or methicillin-resistant staphylococcus aureus, is probably the most common multi-drug resistance, which leads to high death and illness rates. These bacteria have become immune to drugs that normally cure it, making it harder to treat.

Other Causes of Drug and Antibiotic Resistance

These bacteria strains and their infections develop drug resistance through extensive antibacterial drug use. Natural evolution also helps them develop resistance. Besides overuse, antibacterial resistance evolves naturally. With the help of antibiotics, natural selection helps bacteria eliminate the weaker strains and make more resistant ones. It makes antibiotic drugs less effective.

Antibiotic resistance can also be caused by self-medication. Medication prescriptions based on someone else's advice or a person's initiative have increased the risk of antibiotic resistance. This resistance is more prevalent in areas with inadequate medical response and a history of self-medication.

The public's lack of understanding of antibiotic resistance's combination, administration, and assumptions contribute to the rapid increase in antibiotic-resistant bacteria. Also, factors such as the increased use of antibiotics during the global pandemic, untreated waste from the pharmaceutical industry, improper disposal of expired and unused medications, and giving antibiotics to livestock as growth supplements and preventative measures have contributed to an increase in antibiotic-resistant bacteria and its spread between humans and animals.

Natural Antibiotics

Concerns about the potency and effectiveness of antibacterial drugs have emerged as the number of resistant bacteria species has increased. Synergist antibiotics have been prescribed, but there are still concerns about their use. Natural selection causes multi-drug multi-drug-resistant to evolve and eliminate weaker strains.

Natural antibiotics are a treatment that has been around for a while but only recently reemerged as a focus for research as scientists look for new ways to slow the spread of antibiotic-resistant bacteria and improve their effectiveness.

Regular antibiotics treat bacterial infections, but natural antibiotics are safer alternatives. Natural antibiotics are chemical substances found in plants or natural products with the ability to kill bacteria.

Natural antibiotics are herbs, plants, supplements, and other naturally occurring substances with strong antibacterial properties and can treat bacterial infections. They are recommended instead of regular antibiotics due to fewer side effects and antibacterial properties. Unlike regular antibiotics, they are not synthesized in medical laboratories.

With the advent of synthetic antibiotics, do we really need natural antibiotics? Natural antibiotics serve a simple and effective purpose, which has made them the "go-to solution" for less serious infections. Since laboratory-produced antibiotics are also a driving force behind the rise in antibiotic-resistant infections, finding a solution that negates this advantage has led us back to natural antibiotics use.

Natural antibiotics are easier and less expensive solutions to many health infections. They are also non-synthetic, reducing the risk of resistant bacteria strains developing during or after treatment. They are also used with other antibiotics for treatment and have fewer side effects than synthetic antibiotics.

Antibiotics were not the first-line treatment for bacterial infections until early 1940, when the first antibiotic was developed. Since the pharmaceutical industry recently realized the power of herbs and ingredients, they have been combined with non-natural antibiotics to make phytopharmaceuticals that are stronger than non-natural antibiotics.

Despite promising results, the combination of natural and synthetic antibiotics should not be used without a doctor's prescription. Nowadays, many doctors recommend natural antibiotics over synthetic ones because they provide a more holistic approach to treating bacterial infections. Using natural antibiotics decreases inflammation risks and promotes healthy bacteria growth as opposed to resistant strains. Natural antibiotics strengthen the immune system while combating microbial and parasitic infections.

Instead of treating yourself, it's best to talk to a doctor because some antibiotics and supplements react badly with others.

Antibiotic resistance is on the rise, and new measures to improve human health and combat rising bacteria resistance are required. Combinations of antibiotics have become a viable option after extensive research by the medical and pharmacological communities. Synergy is what we seek in these combinations. Antibiotic synergy occurs when two or more antibacterial medications are combined to treat a disease.

This synergy increases their potency over applying the antibiotics individually. Synergist antibiotics kill bacteria that have become resistant because they have been exposed to antibiotics or due to natural selection. Side effects from antibiotics are manageable with the proper use of synergist antibiotics, which also help reduce the spreading of antibiotic-resistant bacteria and eventually eliminate infectious diseases.

Natural antibiotics are more convenient for treating bacterial infections. These antibiotics, in food, plants, or supplements, are naturally occurring antibacterial chemicals that aid in fighting against bacterial infections. They have fewer side effects, are more widely available, and are less expensive. They combat bacterial infection-related inflammation and prevent the spreading of resistant bacteria.

Mostly, we increase antibacterial resistant infections and decrease the efficacy of synergist antibiotics through self-medication and misinformation. Do not take antibiotics, whether natural or made in a lab, unless a doctor prescribes them; this will help you avoid dangerous interactions or side effects.

Individuals and health professionals must wash their hands frequently to reduce the risk of infection and properly dispose of antibiotics after use or expiration. Individuals should practice good hygiene and incorporate it into their food preparation while avoiding foods grown with antibiotics for disease prevention or growth enhancement. Patients should only use antibiotics prescribed by an accredited healthcare professional, never demand or use an antibiotic deemed unnecessary by the healthcare worker, and never share or re-use leftover antibiotics.

In turn, healthcare workers must only dispense and prescribe antibiotics when necessary and engage in conversation with patients about antibiotic usage, resistance, disposal, and bacterial infection prevention. They should go a step further and report antibiotic-resistant infection cases to policymakers and the healthcare industry's surveillance teams. These efforts are advised to increase the potency and achieve the goal of synergist antibiotics.

Chapter 6

Strengthening the Immune System

The immune system is a complex network of cells, tissues, organs, and the substances they produce that fight infections and foreign substances in the body. White blood cells, lymph nodes, lymphatic veins, and bone marrow make up this system, and they must be powerful and efficient enough to combat major and minor infections.

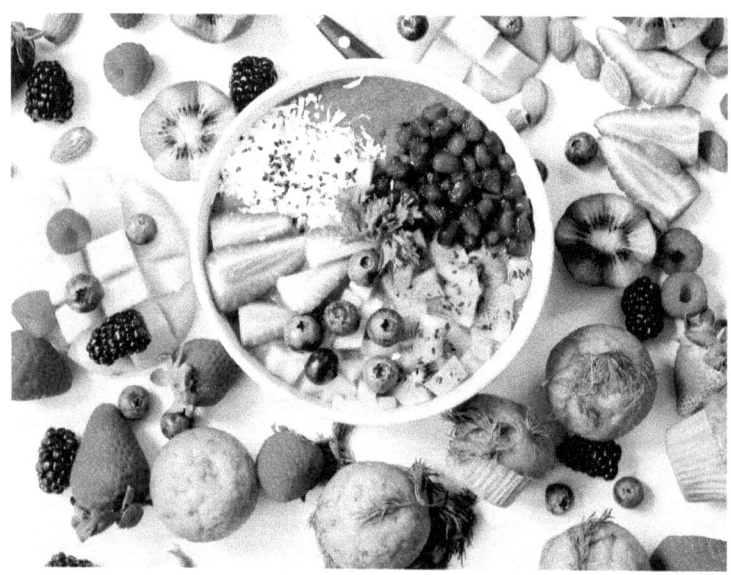

Strengthening the immune system entails taking all necessary precautions to ensure the body's defenses are strong and unharmed to combat infections. Although several pills and products are on the market claiming to boost immunity, maintaining a strong immune system entails more than just ingesting a combination of herbs, vitamins, and minerals.

The immune cells are distinct cells that react to pathogens differently. Due to this, it is particularly difficult to boost the immune system cells. It is a complex system with the potential to develop an autoimmune disorder, which occurs when the immune system is unable to recognize foreign substances and fights against the body's cells, resulting in a great deal of pain and discomfort.

Adhering to basic health recommendations is the best action you can take to naturally maintain a healthy immune function. The first line of defense against any microorganism attack is good health. Every system in the body performs better when it is protected from external irritants and strengthened by healthy lifestyle practices such as regular exercise, eating a balanced diet, avoiding alcohol and smoking, hand washing, stress reduction, adequate rest, and vaccinations. Vaccinations are important because they strengthen the immune system to fight off illnesses before they become serious.

The Importance of Strengthening the Immune System After Using Antibiotics

Antibiotics interfere with the cells of microorganisms in various ways, such as preventing the bacterium from constructing a cell wall, reproducing, or storing and using energy. They eliminate healthy bacteria that help to maintain balance in your body, particularly in the digestive tract, when carrying out these activities. It can negatively impact the body, causing indigestion, vomiting, stomach upset, nausea, diarrhea, and other symptoms. As a result, after taking antibiotics, you should strengthen your immune system to keep your digestive system and overall body function healthy.

Benefits of a Strong Immune System

- Taking steps to strengthen your immune system keeps you healthy. It aids in forming a barrier that prevents infectious substances or antigens from entering your body and infecting you.

- A strong immune system ensures quick recovery from illness and injury. People with higher immune systems recover from injuries faster because their immunity promotes healing, whereas those with lower immunity need more time.

- You are less likely to become tired easily when your immune system is strong. Exercise is one way to boost your immune system and stay active. When you exercise, your body frequently moves, allowing you to maintain a healthy weight, stay active, and feel stronger.

- Contracting a serious disease or illness is uncommon because a strong immune system helps your body fight infections. The defense system produces proteins, white blood cells, and other molecules to attack and eliminate pathogens, which occur mostly before the infection spreads to all parts of the body.

Herbs and Ingredients That Can Be Used to Strengthen the Immune System

Many herbs and ingredients are pathogen-resistant, meaning they effectively combat germs like bacteria, viruses, and worms. Their frequent inclusion in a healthy diet carries a low risk of side effects while increasing the immune system's resistance to illnesses.

The following are a few examples of these herbs and how they help strengthen the immune system:

Echinacea

The Echinacea plant, known as the coneflower, is a member of the Daisy family of flowering plants. The petals are purple or pink, depending on the variety. Echinacea comes in nine widely recognized varieties, but only three have medicinal properties, which are E. Angustifolia, E. pallida, and E. purpurea. It is common in North America and grows in moist to dry wooded areas. This herb has a wide range of applications. It has antiviral and antioxidant properties and properties that help reduce inflammation and pain.

As a result, echinacea is an excellent herb for boosting and supporting your immune system. It accomplishes this by activating and releasing cytokines via macrophages and other intrinsic immune system cells. Following echinacea treatment, immune cells exhibit increased phagocytic activity and foreign particle uptake.

Elderberry

The dark purple elderberry, botanically known as Sambucus nigra, is a fruit grown on European elder trees. It has long been used to treat colds and flu. Due to its antifungal, antimicrobial, and antibacterial properties, elderberry is commonly used to produce many supplements. It aids in strengthening the body's defense system and contains various immune-boosting antioxidants, including vitamins A, B, and C. These vitamins and antioxidants help you maintain a healthy immune system and fight illnesses like flu and the common cold.

Elderberry also contains anthocyanins, a chemical compound with antioxidant properties that give berries their black, red, purple, or blue coloration. They are believed to prevent flu viruses from multiplying within our bodies, which delay or shorten the flu's symptoms.

Garlic

Garlic, also known as Allium sativum, is a perennial plant related to the onion and belongs to the Allium genus. Garlic improves white blood cell effectiveness and strengthens immune function, in addition to improving food flavor. It has antibacterial, antiprotozoal, and antiviral properties, allowing it to help prevent respiratory and chest infections and treat the common cold.

Allicin is a garlic compound that can kill bacteria causing food poisonings, such as salmonella and E. coli. Since it also aids digestion, it is used to treat intestinal worms and parasites.

Reishi

Reishi's botanical name is Ganoderma lucidum, known as lingzhi or spiritual mushroom in China. It grows naturally near the bases and trunks of deciduous trees, especially maples. Although wood chips, hardwood logs, and sawdust can also be used to grow it. Reishi is classified as an adaptogen because it promotes a healthy stress response and aids in balancing numerous body systems and organs.

These mushrooms contain beta-glucans, which activate immune system cells such as monocytes, lymphocytes, and dendrites. When these cells are stimulated, they improve their ability to recognize and attack infections. Reishi is available in pill and powder form.

Fire Cider

Due to its medicinal properties, fire cider is a potent beverage known as a master tonic. Some ingredients used to make fire cider include apple cider vinegar, honey, vinegar-marinated garlic, ginger, onion, horseradish, spicy peppers, and other immune-boosting and flavorful ingredients like turmeric. Fire cider is effective because it contains several herbs that work together to clear the sinuses and fight infections. You can make a bottle of it and take a shot whenever you feel a cold coming on, sprinkle some on your salad every night, or add some to your quinoa or rice.

Ginseng

Ginseng refers to varieties of small, slowly growing plants with fleshy roots, a medium-sized stem, oval-shaped green leaves, and a light-colored forked root. Ginseng can enhance and restore health.

Since extreme long-term stress can compromise your innate immunity, you need a healthy HPA axis to manage stress's impact effectively.

This plant supports the hypothalamus, pituitary, and adrenal axis, which regulate how the immune system responds to stress. Ginseng can also promote a healthy immune response by influencing immune cells such as B cells, T cells, and macrophages, which recognize and neutralize threats to the body. Due to its potency, you should consult with a specialist before incorporating it into your routine. Ginseng can be consumed by taking ginseng capsules or brewing ginseng tea with fresh ginseng root.

Andrographis

Andrographis paniculata, a member of the Acanthaceae family, is found primarily in Southeast Asia, including India and Sri Lanka. Andrographis paniculata leaves have primarily been used to maintain healthy levels of immune cells in the blood and normal body temperature. In Ayurveda and traditional Chinese culture, Andrographis is known as the "King of Bitters" and is traditionally used to promote a healthy gastrointestinal system and microbiological flora, which are required for a healthy defense system.

Astragalus

Astragalus root, known as Huang Qi in Traditional Chinese Medicine, boosts immunity and resilience to sporadic physical and emotional stressors. This plant boosts the immune system while also assisting the body in adjusting to daily stress. Polysaccharides, which are complex carbohydrates in astragalus, influence the microflora and immune function of the gastrointestinal tract. Additionally, astragalus supports the health of mucous membranes and intestinal epithelial cells, which, in turn, supports immunological activity in the respiratory system.

Ginger

Ginger is a spicy herb that grows in tropical areas and is one of the most commonly eaten aromatic plants. Ginger root, Zingiber officinale, supports a healthy immune response by aiding digestion and blood circulation. Gingerols and shogaols are pungent substances found in ginger root that aid blood flow and benefit the entire body. Its anti-inflammatory and antioxidant properties help improve immune function. When feeling chilly, nothing beats a hot cup of ginger tea with lemon and honey.

Goldenseal

The eclectics, Native Americans, learned about this plant in the nineteenth century. The goldenseal root is a naturally occurring source of the recently popular berberine. This herb strengthens and supports the mucous tissues of the respiratory and gastrointestinal tracts and the digestive process. Two of the alkaloids found in goldenseal are hydrastine and berberine, which boost immune function. It is antimicrobial because it kills microorganisms and potentially inhibits cancer development.

Grindelia

Grindelia robusta is a member of the Asteraceae family. Grindelia is a Native American plant commonly used to support the respiratory system and relieve inflammation in the respiratory tract. This plant promotes the health of the mucus layer in the respiratory tract. Modern herb specialists use grindelia, whose blossoms emit sticky syrup to strengthen the lungs and surrounding tissue. It also possesses antibacterial properties, resulting from the actions of the saponosides and polyphenols in it. In addition, it possesses antioxidant and anti-inflammatory properties.

Maitake

The Maitake mushroom, known as Grifola frondosa, is a fungus that grows indefinitely on hardwoods. It is highly valued in Japanese and Traditional Chinese Medicine for immune system support. In Japanese medicine, it is known as the Hen of the Woods, and chefs adore it for its earthy flavor and delicate texture. Like their cousin Reishi, the fruiting bodies of maitake mushrooms contain beta-glucans and are frequently used to support overall body health. It boosts the immune system by providing maximum cellular support.

Olive Tree

The olive tree, scientifically known as Olea Europea, was revered by the ancient Egyptians and Greeks as a symbol of wisdom, peace, and longevity. It has long been regarded as a sacred plant. Although olive oil and olives are popular for skin care and hair growth, olives also provide antioxidant support. They promote normal body temperature and immune cell levels, which improves immunological and cardiovascular health.

Oregano

Origanum vulgare, more commonly known as oregano, is referred to as "the joy of the mountain" in Greek. Due to its powerful volatile oils, oregano has a long history of supporting healthy immune responses and being a natural antioxidant source promoting normal respiratory function. Also, it has been utilized in the kitchens of Europe for millennia.

Basil

Basil is a beautiful herb from India that has been used for hundreds of years in Traditional Chinese Medicine and Ayurvedic treatment. Basil has many health benefits, including strengthening the immune system, slowing the aging process, and fighting bacteria. Additionally, it inhibits cancer cell growth and fights diabetes. It has a high vitamin content and is used as a topping for salads and other foods.

Kakadu Plum

According to reports, the Kakadu plum has the highest vitamin C content of any edible plant, and vitamin C is one of the nutrients beneficial to the immune system. It also contains ellagic acid, minerals, and polyphenols, which are high in antioxidants. According to professionals, when applied topically, Kakadu plum extracts significantly improve skin hydration and suppleness while reducing pigmentation, redness, and dark spots on the body.

It is well known for promoting the body's natural production of procollagen and hyaluronic acid, which protect the skin from UV rays and free radical damage. Moreover, it has strong anti-inflammatory properties that promote collagen synthesis, reduce hyperpigmentation, and can treat open wounds and sunburns.

Neem

Neem is a natural herb derived from the Azadirachta indica tree, known as Indian lilac and Azadirachta indica. The extract is made from the tree's seeds and has had prolonged use in history. Neem is well known for its pesticide and insecticide properties and its use in hair and dental treatments.

It is used in granola production and other healthy foods and supplements. It can be applied topically.

According to research, neem protects against insects, germs, viruses, malaria, and microorganisms. Due to its effectiveness against mosquitos, it has potent anti-inflammatory, antibacterial, and anti-malarial properties. It is a powerful antioxidant, removing free radicals and contributing to the emergence of certain diseases.

Peppermint

Dried or fresh peppermint is known as Mentha piperita leaves. Although peppermint originated in Europe, it is now grown worldwide. Peppermint is a scented herb made by combining spearmint and watermint. In addition to its medical use, it is used as a flavoring or fragrance additive in food, toothpaste, mouthwash, and other products. Peppermint helps improve digestive health, is beneficial in preventing illness, and boosts the immune system by increasing key humoral immune markers and improving growth performance.

Rooibos Tea

Rooibos tea is known as red tea and red bush tea. The leaves of the Aspalathus linearis shrub, commonly grown on South Africa's western coast, are used to make the tea. The leaves are fermented to make traditional Rooibos, giving them a reddish-brown hue. Although green Rooibos, which have not been fermented, are also available. It is usually more expensive than regular tea, has a grassier flavor, and contains more antioxidants. Rooibos tea is typically consumed unflavored or sweetened.

Iron, calcium, vitamin D, potassium, copper, zinc, manganese, magnesium, and alpha hydroxyl acid are among the antioxidants and nutrients in Rooibos. It is an effective treatment for allergies like hay fever and allergy-related bronchitis. Rooibos extract also has anti-aging properties because it reduces the impact of oxidative byproducts on cerebral pathways, promoting concentration and lowering stress. Furthermore, bioflavonoids, which increase blood circulation, lower blood pressure, and prevent hemorrhaging, have been found in Rooibos extract, making it useful for boosting the cardiovascular system.

Rosemary

Along with oregano, thyme, lavender, and basil, rosemary is a member of the Lamiaceae, which is a mint family. The herb is high in calcium, iron, and vitamin B6 and adds a pleasant flavor to dishes like chicken and lamb. Unlike teas and liquid extracts, which are frequently made from fresh or dried leaves, it is typically prepared as a whole dried herb or a dried powdered extract. Several rosemary-containing products are available for purchase online.

The herb has been revered for its healing properties since ancient times. It relieves joint pain, improves memory, boosts the immune and circulatory systems, and promotes hair growth. Rosemary has many chemicals that fight inflammation and free radicals and is known to help strengthen the immune system and improve blood circulation.

Organic Sage

The sage plant's body is thin, and its leaves are furry. The wiry stem grows to about a foot in height and has oblong leaves paired and rounded at the ends. Both sides of the leaf have distinct veins that are slightly wrinkly. This herb thrives in locations with plenty of sunlight and good drainage. Most sage species can survive the winter but must be maintained regularly.

Organic sage's natural antibacterial, preservative, and bacteria-killing properties are well known in the meat industry.

Organic sage contains the phenolic flavonoids apigenin, diosmetin, luteolin, and volatile oils like rosmarinic acid, which are easily absorbed by the body. With its long history of medicinal use, it has treated numerous ailments, including respiratory issues and stomach disorders. Sage has been shown to have antibacterial, antioxidant, anticancer, anti-free radical, and anti-inflammatory properties that protect the body from many diseases.

Ginko

The leaves of the Ginkgo biloba tree are shaped like fans. The greens are frequently included in supplements and taken orally to treat various ailments. It is commonly taken orally for memory and thought problems, vision problems, anxiety, and numerous other disorders. However, the majority of these applications lack strong scientific support.

The leaves of this well-known shrub contain potent antioxidants that help protect your body from free radical damage. This herb protects the skin from various harmful radiation. Ginkgo extracts, tested on lab rats, potentially reduce brain damage, though it is unknown whether this effect extends to humans.

Citrus Fruits

Citrus fruits are high in vitamin C and include oranges, grapefruit, lemons, limes, clementines, tangerines, etc. These fruits are common in most countries and benefit the immune system. Vitamin C aids in the recovery of colds and other flu-like symptoms.

Citrus fruits aid in the production of white blood cells, which are responsible for attacking foreign bodies and infectious organisms in the body. Since the body does not produce vitamin C like other vitamins, humans must consume citrus fruits or other natural herbs that produce vitamins daily. Adult women should consume 75mg of vitamin C daily, while men should consume 90mg.

Broccoli

Broccoli is an edible flower that grows in large quantities. The stalks and flower florets are eaten cooked and raw and have a cabbage-like flavor. Broccoli is scientifically known as Brassica oleracea italica and is commonly found in the Mediterranean.

Since the Roman Empire, it has been a highly valued food by the Italians. It was first introduced to England in the middle of the 18th century, known as Italian asparagus. Broccoli is high in minerals and vitamins C, A, and E. It is high in fiber and antioxidants. These components contribute to its ability to fight microorganisms and strengthen the immune system.

Almond

Prunus dulcis, or almond, is a Rosaceae family edible seed. It is indigenous to Southwestern Asia. It can be eaten raw, roasted, or blanched. Its use is widespread in the baking and skin care industries. Almonds are high in fat, protein, calcium, iron, phosphorus, and various vitamins.

Almond vitamins and minerals are powerful antioxidants that help boost the immune system. A half cup of almond nuts can provide an adult with all of the vitamins and antioxidants they require each day.

The immune system is a vital body component that should not be overlooked. It is very simple to maintain because all you have to do is live a healthy lifestyle. However, if you want to incorporate any of these herbs into your diet, consult your doctor first to ensure they won't cause an allergic reaction or interfere with your current medications. You must seek medical attention if you feel ill.

Chapter 7

Herbal Medicine Making Handbook

Trees, plants, and grasses are abundant around us, which could explain why we don't value them highly. Aside from their nutritional value, these plants have many medicinal benefits that, when used correctly, can keep you healthy and strong all year, every year. Herbal medicine is also known as phytomedicine and botanical medicine. This medicine, using berries, plant seeds, leaves, roots, flowers, or bark, has been practiced for centuries and can be traced back to early civilization. More specifically, the first written record of herbal medicine use was over 5,000 years ago, during the Sumerian civilization. However, archaeological evidence from cave paintings and fossil discoveries indicate that the use of herbs as medicine dates back 60,000 years in Iraq.

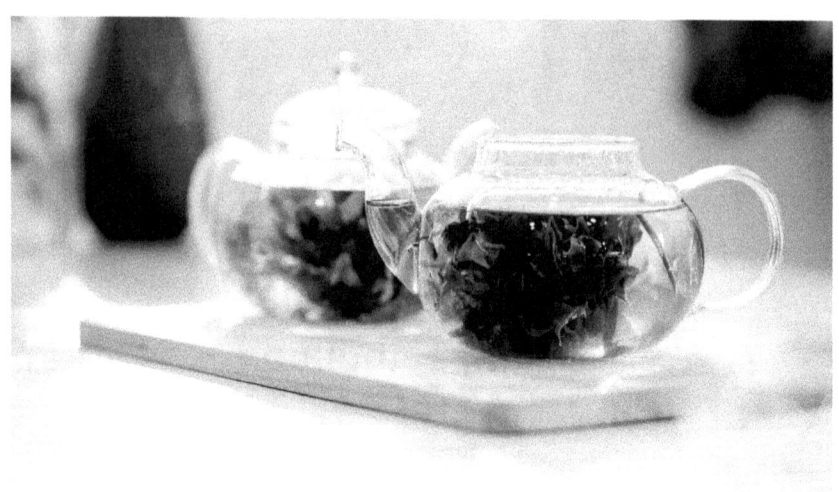

Making Medicine Using Herbs

For many years, men have used herbs to treat their ailments. This knowledge has been passed down from generation to generation, from knowing which plants to use as medicine to how to grow and prepare them. These will be discussed in depth.

Making herbal medicine begins with understanding which herbs are required. This necessitates extensive research to determine the following:

- What illnesses are common in your community or your household?
- What herbs are needed to treat these ailments, and how frequently should they be used?
- How do you grow these herbs?
- At what stage of the herb's development do we use it to make medicine?

- How are these herbs processed or turned into medicine?
- What forms do the end products take - solid, granules, syrup, liquid, etc.?
- What precautions do you take when planting, nurturing, or preparing them?

Importance of Using Herbs as Medicine

Over time, humans have come to rely on certain plants in the environment for medicinal purposes. Some people only use herbs, while others combine their herbal knowledge with their doctors' prescriptions. Ultimately, there are several advantages to using herbs as medicine. Among them are the following:

- **Accessibility and Affordability**

Herbs are all around us and easy to obtain. They have the potential to save us a significant amount of money when used properly. Most medicinal herbs are plants that are usually overlooked or taken for granted due to their abundance.

- **Normalizes the System**

Unlike prescription drugs, herbs in our environment interact with the human system like food while effectively treating various ailments. Including a sufficient amount of carrots in your meal, for example, ensures a daily supply of nutrients, improving your vision and strengthening your immune system.

- **Fewer Side Effects**

Herbs have fewer side effects on the body than synthetic drugs because they occur naturally. In addition, they perform the functions of food and drugs within the body at the same time. Consequently, your system treats them like food while they act as a drug.

Dangers of Using Herbs as Medicine

Despite their benefits and low cost, several risks are associated with using herbs as medicine. They are as follows:

- **Lack of Proper Dosage**

Most herbal medicines are not measured or tested in a laboratory and have no recommended dosages. Furthermore, there is always a risk of overdosing or underdosing because there are no checks and balances when using herbal drugs, especially when homemade.

- **Drastic Side Effects**

Due to how they interact with the human system, there might be a few cases of severe side effects. Additionally, because some of these herbs have not been exhaustively tested on animals or in labs, they pose a significant risk if the side effects become fatal. Gingko Biloba, for example, causes bleeding, which can lead to hemorrhage if not treated promptly.

- **Interaction with Other Drugs**

Doctors frequently advise their patients against using herbs while taking prescribed medications to avoid interactions because herbs do not always go well with prescription drugs. Ginseng, for example, adversely interacts with Warfarin, and the effects on the human system can be severe.

Common Ailments Around You

Every ecosystem has its atmospheric conditions affecting everything in it, including humans. However, certain diseases are indeed caused by environmental factors. It could be due to a dirty environment caused by an unsanitary lifestyle or environmental pollution caused by the emission of harmful substances into the atmosphere, radiation, water contamination, toxic chemical exposure, inadequate sanitation, and air pollution. The local climate influences the spreading of certain diseases. For example, each of the world's major climates, including tropical, desert, Savannah, Mediterranean, temperate, and polar, has distinct diseases. It is your responsibility to determine which is prevalent around you or within your family if a hereditary condition exists. This information will assist you in effectively planning and preparing your herbal medicine to combat them.

Malaria, cough, catarrh, cholera, sinusitis, pneumonia, tuberculosis, asthma, allergy, high blood sugar, and cholesterol can be treated with readily available herbs.

Precautions When Choosing Herbal Medicine

Despite being natural, herbal medicines can have serious side effects if used incorrectly. They can also counteract the effects of conventional medicines, so consult your doctor before deciding which to take.

The following are some precautions to take when using herbal medicines:

- **Self-Education**

You must research the herbs you intend to grow or use as medicine. This research should include reading extensively about them, consulting your doctor or an herbal supplement specialist for advice, and testing the herbs in small quantities to determine how well they work in your system.

- **Proper Observation**

When you first take herbal medicines, pay close attention to changes in your system, whether positive or negative; this will help you decide whether or not to continue using them. Some reactions are mild, while others are severe. If you experience side effects or allergic reactions, discontinue use and consult a doctor.

- **Follow Instructions**

It is critical to follow the instructions or recommendations provided by the manufacturer when using herbal supplements. Read the product label and follow the dosage specifications to determine whether it contains active ingredients you might be allergic to.

- **Avoid Substitution**

You will be tempted to use herbal medicine instead of prescription medications. Do not give in without first seeking medical advice. Herbal medicines are frequently used as supplements, assisting your body's system to perform its normal functions. However, when your body requires prescription drugs to treat certain ailments, you must obtain them. So, don't self-medicate because it could worsen your health.

- **Environmental Considerations**

Quality control varies by country, so what is approved in one country possibly is not approved in another. Herbs used in one country might not be as effective or safe in another. Consequently, you must figure out what works best for you. Herbal supplements are generally classified as food, so they are not as strictly regulated as prescription medications. Therefore, you owe it to yourself to consider where these herbal products are made and how effective they could be.

Herbs for Combating Diseases

Herbs come in different forms, which should be considered when planting, tending, preparing, storing, using, and dosing them. These herbs are classified as Roots, Shrubs, Leaves, and Sap for ease of identification.

- **Roots**

Autumn, which lasts from September to October, is when the roots of various herbs are at their most potent. During this period, energy is concentrated on the roots, and nutrients are channeled downward to them, making it a good time to harvest roots. Some herbal roots used medicinally are as follows:

- Carrots (Daucus carota) are high in vitamin A. They contain other nutrients that, when combined, make a potent herbal medicine.

- Ginger can help with nausea, motion sickness, vomiting, and other symptoms.
- Garlic reduces the risk of heart disease by lowering blood cholesterol levels.
- Dandelion (Taraxacum officinale) and Burdock (Arctium lappa) aid in eliminating germs, normalizing urine flow, reducing fever, and cleansing blood vessels.
- Echinacea (Echinacea purpurea) is an herbal remedy that can treat boils, herpes, and fever. It strengthens blood cells and helps the immune system fight diseases.
- Elecampane (Inula helenium) is useful for bronchitis, asthma, intestinal worms, and other ailments.
- Ginseng is an aphrodisiac and a tonic. It also helps to boost the immune system.
- Valerian is used to treat migraines, fatigue, insomnia, and stomach cramps.
- Turmeric improves memory, fights inflammation, prevents heart disease, and inhibits the growth of cancerous cells.
- Goldenseal treats eye problems, diarrhea, and skin irritations.
- Shrubs

Shrubs serve medicinal and aesthetic purposes, so you can plant them around your home and use them to make herbal medicines as needed. Here are a few examples of medicinal shrubs:

- Elderberry (Sambucus nigra or Canadensis) is used as a food supplement because it helps build the immune system and fights colds and flu.

- Rose of Sharon (Hibiscus syriacus) lowers blood pressure and contains vitamin C and other antioxidants.

- Oregon Grape (Mahonia aquifolium) treats skin issues such as scaly skin, itching, eczema, stomach upset, etc.

- Chaste Tree (Vitex agnus-castus) treats menstrual cycle conditions, menstrual pains and cramps, and menopause-related symptoms.

- Witch Hazel (Hamamelis spp.) treats hemorrhoids, skin diseases, sore throats, and inflammation.

- Willow (Salix spp.) aids in treating lower back pain, osteoarthritis, headaches, and other conditions.

- Hawthorn (Crataegus spp.) reduces cholesterol, blood pressure, and heart disease.

- Rose (Rosa spp.) stimulates the body's natural collagen production, which aids in maintaining healthy skin, hair, and nails.

- Raspberry (Rubus idaeus) lowers blood pressure and improves heart function by providing potassium to the body.

- Douglas Fir (Pseudotsuga menziesii) has antiseptic properties and treats wounds and other skin issues such as burns, cuts, and scrapes.

- Hop Vine (Humulus lupulus) is a relaxant to treat anxiety, insomnia, tension, and attention deficit disorder.
- Lavender (Lavandula angustifolia) improves sleep, is beneficial for skin disorders, promotes hair growth, and is a natural pain reliever.
- Marshmallow (Althaea Officinalis) is used for treating coughs and infections.
- Lemon Balm can help you relax by reducing stress, easing anxiety, improving sleep, and increasing your appetite.
- Peppermint regulates digestion and improves concentration.
- Common yarrow (Achillea millefolium) treats irritable bowel syndrome (IBS) symptoms, such as diarrhea, constipation, and bloating.
- Leaves

Some trees' leaves have medicinal properties. Once mature, these leaves can be used in a variety of ways. They could be massaged into the affected area or made into ingestible substances. Some medicinal leaves are as follows:

- Thyme has antioxidant properties that aid in the fight against fungus and bacterial infections.
- St. John's Wort aids in wound healing and relieves menopausal symptoms.
- Sage is good for controlling blood sugar and cholesterol, maintaining oral health, supporting memory and brain

function, and aiding the body's fight against the growth of cancerous cells.

- Melissa improves your mood, protects against depression, and treats skin diseases and Alzheimer's symptoms.
- Chamomile is beneficial for osteoporosis, cancer treatment and prevention, and treating certain skin conditions.
- Calendula relaxes muscles, fights cancer, and prevents heart disease.
- Arnica can treat bruises and swellings caused by surgical procedures or other cuts.
- Sap

This is the fluid derived from an herb's stem or leaves. These fluids are applied directly to wounds or mixed with other substances and administered orally or by other means. The sap is a vital tree derivative. Minerals, antioxidants, enzymes, and other nutrients are abundant in maple, walnut, and birch saps. Pine sap is ideal for homeopathic remedies. The following are some medicinally useful tree saps:

- Maple sap aids digestion, relieving the digestive system of excessive work. It also contains oligosaccharides to aid in improving gut health.
- Pine sap, when chewed, relieves sore throats and colds and aids in healing wounds.

- Birch sap contains a high concentration of minerals, amino acids, proteins, enzymes, vitamins, and antioxidants.
- Walnut Sap is high in enzymes, minerals, and nutrients, which nourish the skin and boost the immune system.

Tools Needed to Manage Your Herb Garden

Finding the right tools for your herb garden will save you time, energy, and other valuable resources. Keep your tool selection simple for ease of use. Choose sharp, long-lasting, and use high-quality tools. Also, clean and maintain them regularly to ensure they last.

Here are some essential tools for maintaining and managing an herb garden:

Hand Trowel

This tool has a pointed edge and a nearly flat surface for scraping soil off the ground or digging shallow holes. You can use it to scoop up the soil before planting your seed or shrub, and then cover the seed or shrub with the soil you scooped up.

Shovel

Hand trowels are similar to shovels in size. However, shovels have a larger surface area and a longer handle for scooping larger quantities of soil. Shovels are available in various sizes and shapes and are useful for digging deeper holes. They're used to plant or harvest tubers and excavate large areas of land for farming and construction purposes.

Pruning Shears

This is a handy tool resembling a pair of scissors. It is used to cut and trim plants, prune trees to remove extra leaves and stems, and harvest shrubs. Your pruning shears must have very sharp edges to avoid unnecessary tears on your plants as you use the tool, resulting in faster healing of your plants after pruning or cutting.

Watering Can

An ideal watering can has a nozzle with perforations allowing water to be sprayed on plants and crops. This tool makes it easier to water small areas.

Wheelbarrow

This is the main tool for transporting items around the garden. It is used to transport garden tools, water, soil, etc. Since it is operated manually, avoid damaging the herbs while pushing them around the garden.

Gardening Knife

This knife has a more durable blade and handle than a kitchen knife. It is designed to withstand the pressure exerted on the shrubs when being cut. The gardening knife is used to harvest vegetables and other shrubs with thin stems. Some gardening knives have serrated edges to aid in cutting, while others are calibrated to assist in measuring soil depth.

Gardening Gloves

Gloves are essential because they protect your hands from cuts and injuries, keeping them safe. Wearing gardening gloves will help keep your hands clean and germ-free while working in your garden.

Rake

This is a multi-toothed, long-handled tool used to clean up leaves in the garden, whether they were dropped by accident or cut down intentionally. The rake's design removes dead leaves and grasses without disturbing the soil.

Garden Hoe

The garden hoe has a large surface like a shovel and a curve at the head where the wooden or iron handle is fixed. It is used for various tasks, such as digging up the soil to plant roots, making ridges, harvesting roots, and clearing grasses.

Water Tank and Hose

These are required for a long-term water supply to your garden. Having enough water for your garden keeps you calm no matter the state of the weather. The hose is attached to a sprayer and connected to the tank. You can direct the water around the garden when you open the nozzle. The sprayer assists in releasing water in small or large amounts on the herbs, depending on your settings and calibration.

Why You Should Have a Herb Garden

Growing your garden, as stressful as it is, has numerous advantages. The most popular is that your herbs and fruits come fresh from your farm. It is your responsibility to use natural fertilizers rather than chemicals that could be harmful to your system. Growing your garden provides you with the time and opportunity to study the plants, allowing you to expand your knowledge. These advantages are discussed in detail below:

Varieties in Every Meal

Growing your garden ensures you have a variety of herbs to choose from when cooking. Every kitchen time allows you to experiment with various meals and natural ingredients. At the same time, your choice of herbs and spices for your meal can be determined by your family's current health needs, and you will always have what you need.

To Enhance Learning

Your herb garden serves as a research lab where you can try new ideas with herbs. You can try new recipes and gardening techniques with your garden or teach your kids about specific herbs.

Aids in Relaxation

A garden has relaxing effects on the body, affecting how your mind functions. An herb garden serves as a relaxant for your mind, in addition to its medicinal purposes. You can always spend some leisure time in your garden, either working or simply admiring nature's splendor.

For Commercial Purposes

When you plant an herb garden, you grow plants that could be sold commercially. There is a good chance you will grow more herbs than you use. It is up to you to decide whether you want to sell the extra items or give them away to family, friends, and neighbors.

When to Avoid Herbal Medicine

There are times when it is best to avoid using herbal medicine. Below are a few reasons:

When Taking Other Medicines

As previously stated, it is best not to combine herbal medicine with prescription medications or other drugs. Some of the active ingredients in prescription drugs might adversely interact with those in herbal medicine, and these interactions could be harmful to your system or cause allergic reactions.

If You Have Serious Health Conditions

Those with liver or kidney disease, or similar conditions, are advised to avoid using herbal medicine unless prescribed by their doctors. Even in this case, you must strictly adhere to the instructions and recommendations provided. These serious health conditions can be exacerbated by regularly using herbal medicines, and the damage might not be apparent until it is too late.

When Expecting Surgery

It is strongly advised to refrain from using herbal medications if you are scheduled for surgery. Your health and medical history will be requested before the surgery, including information on medications you have recently taken. It will be difficult to thoroughly analyze herbal medicines in your medical history because most herbal medicines do not list the active ingredients.

When Pregnant or Breastfeeding

Whatever you take while pregnant or nursing goes to your baby. Avoid using herbal medicines if you fall into these categories for your child's well-being.

Elderly and Children

Older people have feeble organs that cannot process the active ingredients in herbal medicines due to their age. The same is true for children, whose organs aren't fully developed to help with the digestion and metabolism of these herbal substances. Consequently, it is best to avoid giving herbal medicines to anyone in these categories and seek medical advice if necessary.

Making medicine from herbs can be enjoyable and educational. It also includes some exciting challenges, more likened to an adventure into the world of herbs and plants' endless possibilities. Although these herbs have numerous applications, they have not been tested in an official laboratory to confirm their active ingredients, uses, efficacy, side effects, and other vital information. Therefore, they are not widely recommended by health practitioners, and you should always seek your doctor's advice before using them. Since some of these herbs might negatively interact with your prescribed medications, always consult your doctor before taking them or adding new ones to your list of food supplements. For example, valerian roots can significantly impact how sedatives work in our bodies. If you are pregnant or breastfeeding, avoid using herbal supplements. Furthermore, suppose you care for older people or children. In that case, it is best not to give them herbal medicines because their systems might be too weak to handle their digestion and metabolism (as in the case of an elder) or have not matured sufficiently (as in the case of a child).

Proper information about the herbs you use or intend to use must be obtained. Thorough research will allow you to prepare for any eventuality long before it occurs and avoid and prevent what you can. Having your own herb garden will enable you to teach your family about these herbs and encourage you to try as many different combinations as your creative mind can think of. Moreover, you should have the proper tools and equipment to care for and manage your herb garden.

Chapter 8

Herbal Antibiotic Recipes I

Herbal antibiotics are a potent and effective option for natural remedies. They help fight infection and boost your immune system to make you less likely to get sick in the first place.

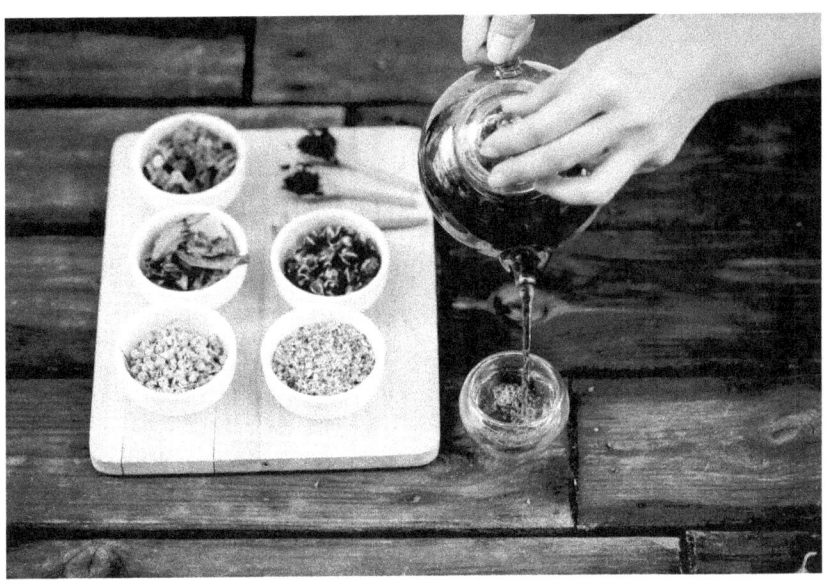

Many different herbs can be used as antibiotic agents, each with unique benefits. When choosing an herbal antibiotic remedy, selecting the right combination of herbs for your specific needs is essential.

Do Natural Antibiotics Work?

There is a common misconception that natural remedies are not as effective as traditional medicines. However, this could not be further from the truth. Natural antibiotics have been used for centuries to treat a variety of infections.

Natural antibiotics can also be as effective as their synthetic counterparts. They often contain powerful plant-based compounds that can kill bacteria and other microorganisms.

Herbal antibiotics are often more effective than their synthetic counterparts.

Not only do herbal antibiotics work to kill harmful bacteria, but they also help boost your immune system because many herbs contain potent antioxidants that help fight infection. This is significant because a strong immune system is key to preventing infections.

Many different natural antibiotics are available, each with unique benefits. The most popular include garlic, oregano oil, and Manuka honey.

Herbal Antibiotic Recipes to Keep You Healthy

When fighting infection, few things are more powerful than antibiotics. But before you head to the doctor for a prescription, consider one of these herbal antibiotic recipes. These time-tested remedies can help you feel better fast, from teas to tinctures.

Garlic, Ginger, and Turmeric Paste

Making your ginger, turmeric, and garlic paste is easy and can be done in just a few simple steps. Fresh turmeric root gives the best flavor, but powdered turmeric is just as good. The combination of these three powerful ingredients makes it a potent antibiotic remedy.

Ingredients:

- 1/2 teaspoon of garlic powder
- 1/2 teaspoon of ginger powder
- 1/4 teaspoon of turmeric powder
- 1 tablespoon of coconut oil
- 1 tablespoon of apple cider vinegar

Instructions:

1. Combine the garlic, ginger, and turmeric powders in a small bowl.
2. Add the coconut oil and apple cider vinegar, and mix until everything is well combined.
3. Apply a small amount of the paste to the affected area and cover it with a bandage. Repeat as needed until the infection clears.
4. Leave it for 30 minutes, remove and rinse with warm water.

5. Store the paste in a glass jar in the fridge for up to a month.

6. The paste can also be frozen for up to three months.

Benefits

This flavorful paste is perfect for adding a boost of flavor to any dish, and it's also packed with health benefits. Turmeric is well-known for its medicinal qualities, including as an excellent antiseptic. It is widely used in healing wounds by applying a turmeric paste to the injury. Turmeric is also anti-carcinogenic and boosts immunity, maintain cholesterol levels, aid digestion, and helps regulate metabolism and blood pressure.

Tips

Add honey or black pepper for added benefits. Start with a smaller amount of turmeric and gradually increase as needed if you have a sensitive stomach. Turmeric can stain your skin and clothes, so wear old clothes when using it.

Caution

Turmeric can thin your blood, so if you take blood-thinning medication, please consult your healthcare provider.

Echinacea Tea

Echinacea tea is made by steeping the leaves and flowers of the echinacea plant in hot water. Echinacea is a daisy family member and native to North America. It has been used by Native Americans for centuries as a natural remedy to treat ear infections and pain. Three main echinacea plants are used to make tea: Echinacea pallida, Echinacea purpurea, and Echinacea Angustifolia.

Ingredients:

- 1 teaspoon of dried echinacea flowers
- 1 cup of boiling water
- Honey or lemon (optional)

Instruction:

1. Pour boiling water over the echinacea flowers in a mug.
2. After steeping for 10 minutes, strain the flowers.
3. Add honey or lemon to taste and drink 3 times a day.

Echinacea tea has a tingling, refreshing, and invigorating flavor. Floral notes complement pine needles' sharp freshness and meadowsweet's soft, round taste. Commonly blended with lemongrass and mint, Echinacea tea is a delicious and refreshing beverage.

Benefits

Echinacea tea is an herbal tea made from the leaves and flowers of the plant Echinacea purpurea. This tea has many benefits, including a natural antibiotic, which helps fight infection and speed up recovery. People living with Asthma also benefit from the tea's anti-inflammatory properties.

Tips

When brewing echinacea tea, it's essential to use high-quality loose teas or tea bags for their best flavor. This tea can also be made using fresh or dried echinacea leaves, roots, and flowers. Limit echinacea tea consumption to one to three cups a day to avoid adverse side effects.

Echinacea tea is generally safe to consume, with few side effects. However, some people experience stomach upset or irritation. Pregnant or nursing women should not consume echinacea. Those with allergies to plants in the daisy family should also avoid this tea.

This herbal tea is naturally caffeine-free, so it can be enjoyed all day long.

Caution

Tea made from the Echinacea plant can cause an allergic reaction in some people. Symptoms include itching, swelling of the face, lips, or tongue, and difficulty breathing. If you experience these symptoms after drinking echinacea tea, discontinue use and seek medical attention immediately.

Goldenseal Ointment

Goldenseal is an herbal remedy used for centuries to treat various ailments. The goldenseal plant is a buttercup family member and native to North America.

Ingredients:

- 1 teaspoon of dried goldenseal root
- 1 cup of boiling water
- 1 tablespoon of olive oil or coconut oil
- 1 tablespoon of beeswax

Instructions:

1. Place the goldenseal root in a mug and pour boiling water over it. Allow the tea to steep for 10 minutes, then strain the root.
2. Add the olive oil, coconut oil, and beeswax to a double boiler and heat until the beeswax is melted.
3. Remove from heat and add the goldenseal tea. Stir until well combined.
4. Pour into a glass jar and allow to cool completely before using.
5. Apply it to the affected area once it's cooled.

Benefits

Goldenseal is a plant with many benefits and can be used in different ways. Plant stems (rhizomes) and roots make teas, liquid extracts, capsules, tablets, and natural skincare products.

Goldenseal is a powerful antibacterial herb used to treat numerous infections. The active ingredient in goldenseal, berberine, is a potent antibacterial agent effective against many bacteria. Goldenseal is also rich in other compounds with antibacterial, antifungal, and antiparasitic properties, making it an effective treatment for many different infections.

Goldenseal ointment treats various skin conditions, including eczema, psoriasis, and diaper rash. The balm has antibacterial and anti-inflammatory properties, making it an excellent choice for treating cuts, scrapes, and burns. Goldenseal is a powerful antibiotic herb that helps kill harmful bacteria.

Tips

Goldenseal ointment can be stored in a cool, dark place for up to six months. If you have sensitive skin, test the ointment on a small area of skin before using it on a larger area, or dilute the ointment with water before applying it to your skin.

Caution

Goldenseal is not recommended for pregnant or breastfeeding women. Goldenseal can cause side effects, such as gastrointestinal upset, diarrhea, and vomiting.

Echinacea Tincture

Echinacea tincture is a concentrated extract of the herb echinacea. This extract is made by soaking the dried herb in alcohol or vinegar. The resulting mixture is strained to remove the solid plant matter.

Ingredient:

- Dried echinacea herb
- Alcohol or vinegar

Instructions:

1. Soak the dried echinacea herb in alcohol or vinegar for several weeks.
2. Strain the mixture to remove the solid plant matter.
3. Take a full dropper (25-30 drops) of the tincture 3 times daily.

Benefits

Echinacea tincture is a potent extract of the echinacea herb. This extract has powerful infection-fighting properties and effectively treats several infectious diseases, including herpes, malaria, syphilis, and urinary tract infections. This tincture can be used at the first sign of a cold or flu.

Tips

Use fresh or dried echinacea flowers and roots when making your echinacea tincture. If you are using fresh herbs, clean them thoroughly before starting the tincturing process. The ratio of herb to liquid should be 1:5 for best results.

When using dried herbs, it is best to grind them into a powder before adding them to the liquid. It helps release more of the active compounds into the tincture.

Use a glass jar with a tight-fitting lid when making your tincture to prevent the mixture from spoilage.

Echinacea tincture can be taken internally or applied topically. The usual dosage is 1-2 droppers full three times a day when taking echinacea tincture internally. Dilute the mixture with water and apply it to the affected area if you are using it topically.

Caution

If you are allergic to plants in the daisy family, you should not take echinacea tincture, including ragweed, chrysanthemums, marigolds, and daisies. People with autoimmune diseases like lupus or multiple sclerosis should avoid echinacea tincture.

Oregano Oil

Oregano oil is a potent essential oil extracted from the oregano plant's leaves. This oil has a strong, spicy fragrance and is known for its potent antibacterial and antifungal properties.

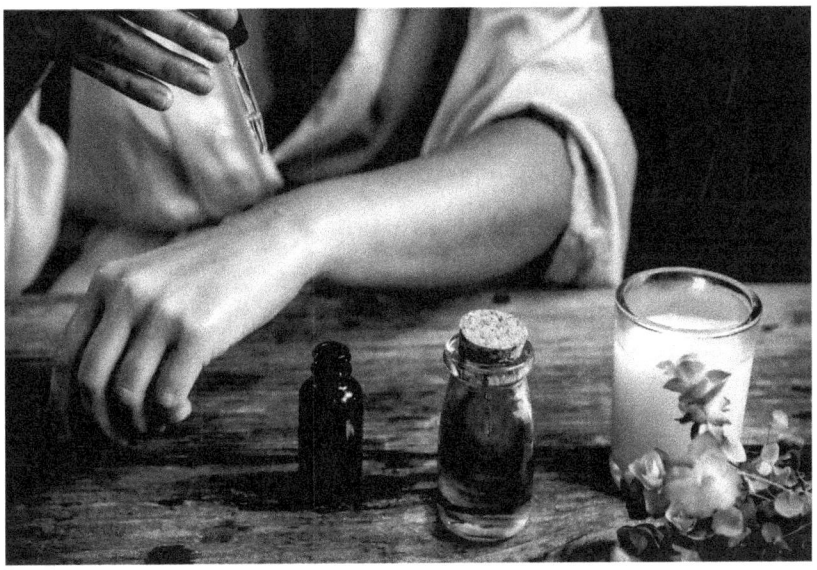

Ingredient:

- 1/2 teaspoon of oregano oil
- 1/4 cup of olive oil

Instructions:

1. Combine the oregano oil and olive oil in a small bowl.
2. Apply the mixture to the affected area.
3. Repeat this process several times a day until the infection clears up.

Benefits

Oregano oil treats various infections, including respiratory infections, urinary tract infections, and skin infections. This oil treats head lice, Candida infections, and stomach ulcers. Oregano oil is a robust antimicrobial agent that can help fight infection and speed the healing process. This oil is also a potent anti-inflammatory agent to reduce swelling and pain.

Oregano oil contains a compound called carvacrol, which has antibacterial and antifungal properties. It is also a powerful antioxidant that boosts your immune system.

Tips

When using oregano oil to treat an infection, it is essential to use a high-quality oil that is 100% pure. This oil can be purchased at health food stores or online.

Caution

Oregano oil is a potent essential oil and should be used with caution. This oil can cause skin irritation in some people. If you experience adverse side effects, discontinue use immediately.

Pregnant women and young children should not use oregano oil. This essential oil can also interact with certain medications, so speak with your healthcare provider before using it.

Rosemary Tea

Rosemary is a fragrant herb with a long history of use in folk medicine. This herb boosts circulation, improves digestion, and relieves pain. Rosemary tea is a delicious way to enjoy the benefits of this herb.

Ingredient:

- 1 teaspoon of dried rosemary
- cup of boiling water

Instructions:

1. Add the dried rosemary to a cup of boiling water.
2. Allow the tea to steep for 5 minutes.
3. Strain the tea and enjoy.

Benefits

Rosemary tea can treat various ailments, including headaches, indigestion, and muscle pain. Besides improving digestion, this tea boosts circulation. Rosemary tea is a soothing beverage that can help reduce stress and anxiety.

Rosemary contains a compound called rosemarinic acid, which has powerful anti-inflammatory and antioxidant properties. This compound helps protect your cells from damage and boosts your immune system.

Tips

Rosemary tea is not recommended for children under the age of 12. If you have a medical condition, consult your healthcare provider before drinking rosemary tea. Do not drink more than 2 cups of rosemary tea a day.

Caution

Rosemary tea is generally safe for most people to drink. Overdosing on rosemary can cause vomiting, seizures, and coma. If you are pregnant or breastfeeding, it is best to avoid rosemary tea.

Marshmallow Root Ointment

Marshmallow root is an herb used for centuries in folk medicine. This herb is known for its ability to soothe and heal the skin. Marshmallow root and leaf supplements are made by extracting compounds from the Althaea Officinalis plant. Marshmallow has many benefits, including natural mucilage, flavonoid antioxidants, and various antibacterial, antiviral, and anti-mucilaginous compounds.

Ingredient:

- 1/4 cup of marshmallow root powder
- 1/2 cup of olive oil or coconut oil
- 1/4 cup of beeswax
- 10 drops of lavender essential oil (optional)

Instructions:

1. Add the marshmallow root powder to a bowl.
2. Pour the olive oil or coconut oil over the powder and stir well.
3. Place the mixture in a saucepan and heat over low heat until it becomes liquid.
4. Remove the pan from the heat and add the beeswax to the mixture. Stir well until the beeswax is melted.
5. Stir in the lavender essential oil (optional).

6. Pour the ointment into a jar and allow it to cool completely before using.

Benefits

Marshmallow root ointment is a soothing and healing ointment. This ointment can help heal wounds, soothe eczema, and reduce inflammation. Marshmallow root ointment can treat sunburns and diaper rash.

Marshmallows are an effective remedy for pain, swelling, and irritation symptoms. It also resolves throat and skin infections, strengthens the gut lining, and prevents permeability.

Tips

You can make this ointment with olive or coconut oil. If you are using coconut oil, use unrefined coconut oil. You can find marshmallow root powder at your local health food store or online.

Caution

Do not use marshmallow root ointment if you're allergic to plants in the Althaea genus. Mucilage-rich plants like marshmallow root can interfere with the absorption of certain medications. So, consult your healthcare provider before using marshmallow root ointment if you are taking medication.

Herbal Sore Throat Gargle

This herbal gargle is a simple, effective way to soothe a sore throat. This gargle can also relieve congestion and fight infections.

Ingredients:

- 1 cup of water
- 1 teaspoon of grated ginger
- 1/2 teaspoon of turmeric powder
- 1 tablespoon of honey
- 1 tablespoon of apple cider vinegar
- 1/4 teaspoon of cayenne pepper (optional)

Instructions:

1. Add the water, ginger, turmeric, honey, apple cider vinegar, and cayenne pepper to a saucepan.
2. Heat the mixture over low heat until it simmers.
3. Remove the pan from the heat and allow the mixture to cool slightly.
4. Gargle with the mixture for a minute and then spit it out.
5. Repeat as needed.

Benefits

This herbal gargle is a soothing and healing remedy for sore throat—honey and apple cider vinegar helps to coat the throat and relieve irritation. Ginger, turmeric, and cayenne pepper are all antibacterial and antiviral herbs that fight infection.

Tips

You can find grated ginger, turmeric powder, and cayenne pepper at your local grocery store or health food store. If you don't have apple cider vinegar, substitute it with white vinegar. You can add a few drops of eucalyptus oil to this gargle to help clear congestion.

Caution

Do not swallow this gargle. Cayenne pepper can cause burning if it gets in your eyes. Do not use this gargle if you're pregnant or have a history of ulcers. If you get the mixture in your eyes, rinse them out with water immediately.

Lemon Balm Tea

Lemon balm (Melissa officinalis) is an herbaceous perennial in the mint family. The leaves have a lemon-like scent and are used to make teas, oils, and ointments. Lemon balm is native to Europe, Central Asia, and Iran but has naturalized in many other countries, including the United States.

Ingredients:

- 1 teaspoon of dried lemon balm leaves or 1 tablespoon of fresh lemon balm leaves
- 1 cup (8 ounces) of boiling water
- Honey or sugar (optional)

Instructions:

1. Pour boiling water over lemon balm leaves.
2. Allow the tea to steep for 3-5 minutes.
3. Strain the tea and add honey or sugar if desired.
4. Enjoy.

Benefits

Lemon balm tea has a range of health benefits. It is particularly effective against candida, which causes digestive problems, brain fog, exhaustion, and more. Lemon balm primarily helps regulate blood sugar levels, but it is not an insulin replacement. In addition, people have been experimenting with lemon balm and found that it helps them battle anxiety.

This herbal tea can treat insomnia and stomach upset. Lemon balm tea is also a great way to boost your mood and fight depression. This tea helps improve your cognitive function and memory.

Lemon balm contains compounds with antiviral, antibacterial, and antifungal properties. This herb also boosts your immune system and fights infections.

Tips

If you are using fresh lemon balm leaves, wash them thoroughly before use. Ginger and mint can also be added to this tea for flavor and health benefits. Use pre-made lemon balm tea bags if you don't have fresh or dried lemon balm leaves.

Caution

Lemon balm is generally considered safe for most people. However, it can interact with some medications. Please speak to your doctor before consuming lemon balm if you are taking any medications. Lemon balm is also not recommended for pregnant or nursing women.

Thyme Tincture

Thyme has a long history of use as herbal medicine. It is especially effective against respiratory infections like bronchitis, whooping cough, and lung congestion.

Ingredients:

- 1 ounce of dried thyme leaves or 2 ounces of fresh thyme leaves
- 1 pint (16 ounces) of vodka or other alcohol
- A dark glass jar with a tight-fitting lid

Instructions:

1. Place the thyme in the jar.
2. Pour the vodka over the thyme, ensuring all leaves are covered.
3. Seal the jar tightly and store it in a cool, dark place for 4-6 weeks.
4. Shake the jar every few days.
5. After 4-6 weeks, strain the thyme leaves from the tincture and discard them.
6. Pour the tincture into a clean glass jar with a tight-fitting lid.
7. Label the jar with the herb's name, the date, and the ratio of herb to alcohol use.
8. Store in a cool, dark place.

Benefits

Thyme tincture is a very effective herbal antibiotic. The antiseptic and antimicrobial properties of thyme make it an effective treatment for skin infections. Thyme tincture is excellent for external use on cuts and scrapes.

Tips

If you are using fresh thyme leaves, wash them thoroughly before use. For added health benefits, add other herbs to this tincture, like garlic or ginger.

Caution

Thyme tincture is potent. It should only be used for a short period, no more than one week. Please consult your doctor if you have any liver problems before using this tincture.

Ginger Tea

Ginger tea is an herbal tea made using ginger root. Ginger tea has many health benefits, including relieving nausea, pain, and inflammation.

Ginger tea is an antibiotic because it contains a compound called gingerol. Gingerol is a phenolic compound with antibacterial activity against Escherichia coli and Staphylococcus aureus.

In addition to its antibacterial properties, ginger tea helps boost your immune system. One study showed that ginger tea increased the production of cytokines, which are molecules that help regulate the immune system.

Ginger tea has a spicy, earthy flavor that some people enjoy. It can be drunk hot or cold and made more or less concentrated depending on personal preference.

Ingredients:
- 1 cup water
- 1-inch piece of ginger root, peeled and sliced
- Honey (optional)

Instructions:
1. Bring the water to a boil.
2. Add the ginger and let steep for 5-10 minutes.
3. Remove the ginger and sweeten it with honey if desired.

Benefits

Ginger tea is a rich source of antioxidants, which are substances that scavenge harmful toxins and byproducts that damage cells. Antioxidants help in preventing chronic diseases like cancer. Ginger's antiviral and antibacterial properties make it effective in fighting infection.

Tips

If you use fresh ginger root, wash it thoroughly before grating or chopping.

You can also buy pre-made ginger tea bags at many stores. The longer you steep the tea, the more concentrated and robust the flavor. If you find the taste of ginger too intense, add a lemon slice to your tea.

Caution

Ginger interacts with certain medications like blood thinners. Consult your healthcare provider before drinking ginger tea if you are taking medications. Possible side effects of drinking ginger tea include heartburn, gas, and bloating.

Hawthorn Berry Tea

Brewing hawthorn berry tea is an ancient practice that dates back over two thousand years. This herbal tea is rich in antioxidants and nutrients, making it a healthy choice for those looking to improve their overall well-being. Hawthorn berry tea offers a range of health benefits, including improved heart health and longevity. These berries grow primarily in Asia and Europe, but their popularity has spread worldwide. Today, you can find hawthorn berry tea, jam, syrup, and wine in many countries.

Ingredients:

- 1 tbsp hawthorn berries dried
- 1 cup water
- Honey optional

Instructions:

1. Add the hawthorn berries to a cup of boiling water.
2. Allow the tea to steep for 5-10 minutes.
3. Strain the hawthorn berries from the tea.
4. Sweeten with honey, if desired.
5. Drink hawthorn berry tea 1-2 times a day.

Benefits

Herbal teas are a great way to improve your health, and hawthorn berry tea is no exception. This recipe harnesses the power of antioxidants and flavonoids to help improve cardiovascular function, ease tension in blood vessels and arteries, and even treat anxiety and stress. So, the next time you feel run down or stressed, brew a cup of this delicious and healing hawthorn berry tea.

Tips

When preparing hawthorn berry tea, it is important to use fresh or dried berries. The tea can be enjoyed hot or cold and is typically sweetened with honey. Some people also add milk or lemon to the tea.

Caution

People with gut problems, heart issues, or on medication should avoid hawthorn berry tea. As always, speak to a doctor before adding any new herb or supplement to your diet.

This tea is not for everyone, but for those it does help, the benefits are great.

Chapter 9

Herbal Antibiotic Recipes II

Peppermint Tea

Peppermint (Mentha Piperita) is a hybrid mint, a cross between watermint and spearmint. The plant, indigenous to Europe and the Middle East, has naturalized in many regions and is now widely distributed throughout the world's temperate zone.

Peppermint tea is naturally caffeine-free and low in calories.

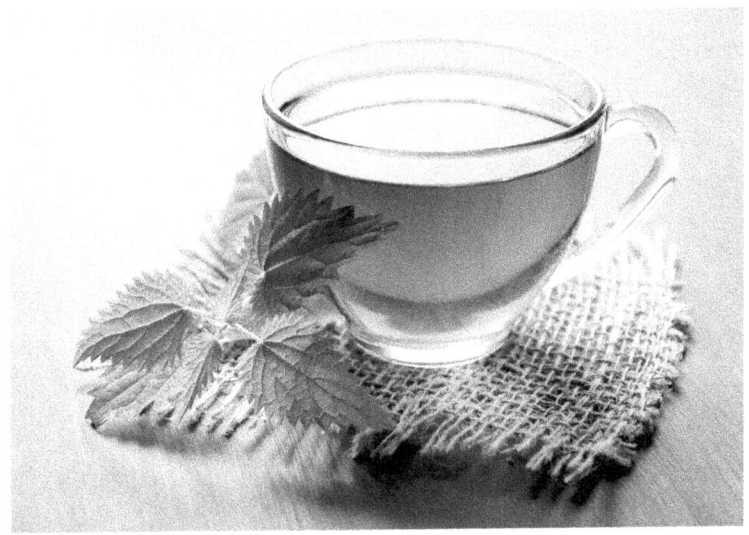

Ingredient:
- 1 teaspoon of dried peppermint leaves
- 1 cup of boiling water

Instructions:
1. Add the peppermint leaves to a cup.
2. Pour boiling water over the leaves and let steep for 5 minutes.
3. Strain the tea and enjoy.

Benefits

Peppermint tea is a refreshing and soothing beverage enjoyed hot or cold. Peppermint tea is also a good source of several nutrients, including vitamin C, manganese, and copper. Peppermint tea is especially beneficial in improving digestion, reducing bloating and gas, and relieving nausea.

The menthol in peppermint has antibacterial and antiviral properties. Peppermint tea can help relieve congestion, coughing, and sore throats.

Tips

If you are not a fan of the peppermint taste, add a bit of honey or lemon to the tea. Add freshly grated ginger to your tea for an extra immune-boosting punch.

Caution

Drinking peppermint tea can cause heartburn and indigestion in some people. Peppermint tea should be avoided if you have GERD or taking medications for heartburn or acid reflux. Peppermint tea interacts with certain medications. If this happens to you, drink the tea with a meal or snacks instead of on an empty stomach.

Eucalyptus Salve

Eucalyptus (Eucalyptus globulus) is a tall, evergreen tree native to Australia. The tree has long been used in traditional medicine for its health benefits.

Eucalyptus oil is steam distilled from the leaves of the eucalyptus tree and has a strong menthol fragrance. The oil is used in various ways, including aromatherapy, massage, and topical application.

Ingredients:

- 1/2 cup of olive oil or coconut oil
- 1/4 cup of beeswax
- 20 drops of eucalyptus essential oil
- 10 drops of peppermint essential oil (optional)

Instructions:

1. Place the olive oil or coconut oil and beeswax in a double boiler.
2. Heat the mixture over low heat, occasionally stirring, until the beeswax is melted.
3. Remove from heat and stir in the eucalyptus and peppermint essential oils.
4. Pour the mixture into a small jar or tin and let cool.
5. Massage a small amount of salve onto the chest and throat as needed.

Benefits

Eucalyptus salve is a topical remedy that can relieve muscle aches and pain, chest congestion, and coughs. When applied to the chest, the salve helps open the airways and makes breathing easier. The eucalyptus essential oil in the salve has antibacterial, antifungal, and anti-inflammatory properties.

Tips

Apply the salve before bedtime for best results, and cover the chest with a warm towel. This will help the body absorb the salve and allow a good night's sleep.

For best results, apply the eucalyptus salve to the chest and throat 2-3 times per day.

Caution

If you are pregnant or breastfeeding, avoid using eucalyptus essential oil. If you have sensitive skin, test the salve on a small area before applying it to a larger area.

Rosemary and Thyme Tea

Rosemary (Rosmarinus officinalis) is an evergreen shrub native to the Mediterranean region. The herb has been used for centuries in cooking and medicine. Rosemary leaves flavor various dishes, including soups, stews, and roasted meats. Rosemary tea is a popular herbal infusion made with fresh or dried rosemary leaves.

Rosemary is also a popular ingredient in cosmetics and personal care products.

Thyme (Thymus vulgaris) is a perennial herb native to the Mediterranean region. The leaves of the thyme plant have a strong, pungent aroma and are used fresh or dried in various dishes. Personal care products and cosmetics also contain thyme.

Ingredients:
- 1 teaspoon of dried rosemary leaves
- 1 teaspoon of dried thyme leaves
- 1 cup of boiling water
- Honey (optional)

Instructions:
1. Place the rosemary and thyme in a cup or mug.
2. Pour the boiling water over the herbs and let steep for 3-5 minutes.
3. Strain the tea and sweeten it with honey, if desired.

Benefits

This delicious and refreshing tea combines the benefits of rosemary and thyme. Rosemary has been used in traditional medicine for centuries to treat headaches, respiratory problems, infections, colds, and stomach ailments.

Rosemary and thyme tea is a great way to boost your immune system and fight infection. Rosemary and thyme's antimicrobial properties help kill bacteria and viruses, making this tea an excellent natural remedy for colds, flu, and other respiratory illnesses.

This tea is also rich in antioxidants, helping protect the body from damage caused by free radicals. Free radicals are unstable molecules that can damage cells and lead to inflammation. Antioxidants help neutralize free radicals and protect the body from damaging effects.

Tips

Rosemary and thyme tea is best enjoyed fresh, but you can also make a larger batch and store it in the fridge for up to 2 days.

If pregnant or breastfeeding, consult your healthcare provider before drinking rosemary and thyme tea.

Caution

Rosemary and thyme tea interact with blood thinners and anticoagulant medications. Consult your healthcare provider before drinking this tea.

Recommendation

Enjoy rosemary and thyme tea 1-2 times daily to fight infection and boost your immune system.

Wormwood Tincture

Wormwood (Artemisia absinthium) is a perennial herb native to Europe, Asia, and Northern Africa. Wormwood is best known for its use in absinthe production, a distilled alcoholic beverage. Wormwood is also used in various bitters and as a flavoring agent in food and beverages.

Ingredients:

- 1 ounce of dried wormwood leaves
- 1 pint of vodka
- Honey (optional)

Instructions:

1. Place the wormwood in a clean glass jar.
2. Pour the vodka over the herb and screw on the lid.
3. Shake the jar well to combine the ingredients.
4. Store the tincture in a cool, dark place for 2-3 weeks.
5. After 2-3 weeks, strain the tincture and discard the herb.
6. Store the tincture in a clean glass bottle and keep it in the fridge.

Benefits

Wormwood tincture is a potent natural remedy for treating various ailments, including digestive problems, respiratory infections, and fevers. The active compounds in wormwood, thujone, and artemisinin, have potent antimicrobial and antiparasitic properties.

Tips

Add a few drops of wormwood tincture to water or juice to help ease digestive problems.

For respiratory infections, take one teaspoon of tincture three times a day.

To treat fevers, take one teaspoon of tincture every hour until the fever breaks.

Caution

Wormwood tincture is not suitable for children or pregnant women. Please speak to your doctor before taking this remedy if you are taking any medications. The ingredient in wormwood is thujone, which is toxic in large doses. Wormwood should only be used under the supervision of a qualified healthcare practitioner.

Chamomile Tea

Most health food stores sell dried chamomile flowers (Matricaria chamomilla) in pre-packaged form. The flowers of the chamomile plant have a sweet, apple-like fragrance and are used fresh or dried to make tea. Chamomile tea is a popular beverage worldwide known for its calming effects. Chamomile tea is made by steeping chamomile flowers in hot water for 3-5 minutes.

Ingredients:

- 1 teaspoon of dried chamomile flowers
- 1 cup of boiling water

Instructions:

1. Place the chamomile flowers in a cup.
2. Pour boiling water over the flowers and let steep for 3-5 minutes.
3. Strain the tea and enjoy.

Benefits

Chamomile tea is a delicious and refreshing way to enjoy the benefits of this fantastic herb. Chamomile has been used for centuries in traditional medicine to treat various ailments, including anxiety, insomnia, and stomach problems. Chamomile tea is a great way to relax and unwind after a long day. Chamomile tea's calming effects also relieve anxiety and promote sleep.

The chamomile flowers contain several compounds, including apigenin and luteolin, which have anti-inflammatory and antioxidant properties. Calcium, magnesium, and potassium are also found in chamomile tea.

Tips

Use fresh or dried chamomile flowers to get the most out of your chamomile tea. Chamomile tea can be enjoyed hot or cold and is best enjoyed without sweeteners.

Caution

Chamomile tea is generally considered safe for most people. However, some people are allergic. If you experience any adverse effects after drinking chamomile tea, discontinue use and consult your healthcare provider.

Clove Bud Oil

Clove bud oil is a natural oil extracted from the clove tree's flower buds. Clove bud oil has a sweet, spicy, and floral aroma and is used in aromatherapy to promote relaxation and well-being. Clove bud oil is known for its antibacterial and antifungal properties.

Ingredients:

- 1 teaspoon of dried clove buds
- 1 teaspoon olive oil

Instructions:

1. Place the clove buds and olive oil in a small bowl.
2. Mix well and apply to the skin.

Benefits

Clove bud oil is an excellent natural remedy for bacterial and fungal infections. The oil has strong antibacterial and antifungal properties that help kill bacteria and fungi. Clove bud oil is also a great way to relieve pain and inflammation. The oil contains compounds, including eugenol and beta-caryophyllene, which have analgesic and anti-inflammatory properties.

Tips

Clove bud oil can be used topically or added to a diffuser for aromatherapy. For topical use, mix the oil with a carrier oil, like jojoba oil or almond oil, before applying it to the skin.

Caution

Clove bud oil can cause irritation and sensitization when used topically. If you experience any adverse effects after using this oil, discontinue use and consult your healthcare provider. Clove bud oil should not be taken internally. Pregnant and breastfeeding women should avoid using this oil.

Elderberry Tea

Elderberry (Sambucus nigra) is a shrub that grows in Europe, North Africa, and Asia. The berries and flowers of the elderberry plant are used to make tea, syrup, jam, and wine. Elderberry tea is a delicious way to enjoy the benefits of this powerful herb.

This herbal tea recipe is simple and can be enjoyed hot or cold. It can be sweetened with honey or stevia to taste.

Ingredient:

- 1/4 cup dried elderberries
- 1 Tbsp fresh grated ginger
- 1 tsp ground cinnamon
- 1 tsp ground cloves
- 1 Tbsp dried orange peel
- 8 cups of water

Instructions:

1. Add all ingredients to a large pot.
2. Bring to a boil, reduce heat, and simmer for 30 minutes.
3. Remove from heat and allow to cool slightly.
4. Pour through a strainer into a pitcher or jar.
5. Enjoy hot or cold, sweetened with honey or stevia to taste.

Benefits

This herbal tea contains elderberries, which are rich in antioxidants and reduce inflammation. Elderberries are also effective in treating colds, flu, and respiratory infections.

Tips

1. Drink 1-2 cups of elderberry tea daily to boost your immune system and fight infection.

2. Store leftover tea in the fridge for up to 5 days.

3. You can find elderberry tea bags at most health food stores.

Caution

Elderberry tea is safe for most people. Consult your healthcare provider if pregnant or breastfeeding.

Herbal Cough Syrup

This homemade cough syrup recipe is a natural way to soothe a cough. Several simple ingredients are used to make the syrup, which is taken as needed.

Ingredients:

- 1/2 cup of honey
- 1/4 cup of apple cider vinegar
- One teaspoon of freshly grated ginger
- 1/4 teaspoon of ground turmeric
- 1/4 teaspoon of ground cinnamon

Instructions:

1. Mix all ingredients in a small jar.
2. Take 1-2 teaspoons as needed.

Benefits

This herbal cough syrup is a delicious and effective way to treat a cough naturally. The honey helps coat the throat and ease coughing, while the vinegar and spices help break up congestion.

The honey, vinegar, and spices in this syrup also have antibacterial and anti-inflammatory properties. Take this syrup as needed to relieve symptoms and feel better quickly.

Tips

To get the most out of this herbal cough syrup, use raw, unpasteurized honey. You can add a squeeze of fresh lemon juice for added flavor and benefits.

Caution

In case of allergy, do not consume this syrup. Start with a small amount of raw honey if you've never taken it before.

Herbal Throat Spray

This herbal throat spray is a great way to soothe a sore throat naturally. It is made with simple ingredients and stored in a small bottle for easy use.

Ingredients:

- 1/4 cup of distilled water
- 1/4 cup of apple cider vinegar
- 1 teaspoon of honey
- 1/4 teaspoon of ground ginger
- 1/8 teaspoon of cayenne pepper

Instructions:

1. Mix all ingredients in a small spray bottle.
2. Spray the back of the throat as needed.
3. Avoid swallowing the spray.

Benefits

This herbal throat spray is an effective way to treat a sore throat naturally. The apple cider vinegar and honey help coat the throat and ease pain, while the ginger and cayenne pepper help break up congestion.

This spray can be used as needed to relieve symptoms and help you feel better fast.

Tips

If you find this throat spray's taste is too strong, add more water to dilute it further. Also, you can use a different vinegar, like white or rice.

Caution

If you are allergic to any of the ingredients in this spray, do not use it. If you have never taken raw honey, start with a small amount to test for allergies.

Yarrow Tincture

Yarrow (Achillea millefolium) is a perennial herb native to Europe and Asia. It has been used for centuries to treat various ailments, including wounds, infections, and colds.

Ingredients:

- 1 cup yarrow leaves and flowers
- 1 cup vodka or other alcohol

Instructions:

1. Harvest yarrow leaves and flowers in the summer when they are in full bloom.
2. Wash them thoroughly to remove any dirt or debris.
3. Place the yarrow in a clean jar, and pour vodka or alcohol over it until the plant material is completely covered.
4. Seal the jar tightly and store it in a cool, dark place for four to six weeks.
5. Shake the pot occasionally to release the yarrow's medicinal properties into the alcohol.
6. Put the tincture in a dark glass bottle after straining it through a coffee filter or cheesecloth.

Apply the tincture to a clean cloth and the affected area. The yarrow tincture can also be taken internally by adding 10-15 drops to water or juice 3 times a day.

Benefit

Yarrow tincture can be used externally or internally. It is most commonly used to treat minor cuts, scrapes, and viral infections like the common cold or flu.

Tips

If you are pregnant or breastfeeding, do not take yarrow tincture internally. You can still use it externally on cuts and scrapes.

Caution

Do not take yarrow tincture if you are allergic to plants in the Asteraceae family, such as chamomile, daisy, or ragweed.

Yarrow tincture is a safe and effective way to treat minor wounds and infections. If you have a more severe disease, see your doctor.

Herbal Drink

Herbal remedies have been used to fight infection for centuries. This herbal drink is a natural antibiotic with plant ingredients known to have antibacterial, antifungal, antiviral, and antiparasitic properties.

Ingredients:

- 15 garlic cloves
- 1/4 cup grated ginger
- 1 whole lemon
- 1/4 cup manuka honey
- 1 Tbsp turmeric powder
- 3 oz apple cider vinegar
- 1 oz olive oil (or 1 tsp coconut oil)
- 1 cup of water

Instruction:

1. Peel and chop the garlic cloves.
2. Grate the ginger root.
3. Squeeze the lemon juice into a bowl.
4. Add all ingredients into a blender and blend until smooth.
5. Pour the mixture into a glass jar with a lid and store in the fridge for up to 2 weeks.

At the first sign of sickness, take a shot of this drink. If needed, you can take an additional four shots of this remedy throughout the day.

Benefit

This herbal drink's combination of ingredients helps fight infection while boosting the immune system. Garlic and ginger have well-known antibacterial properties, while lemon is rich in vitamin C, a nutrient that helps boost immunity. Manuka honey has antimicrobial properties and helps kill pathogens, while turmeric is a potent anti-inflammatory agent. Apple cider vinegar alkalizes the body and fights infection, while olive oil or coconut oil provides essential fatty acids that support the immune system. The key to this remedy is to enhance the immune system's defenses.

This herbal drink is an effective way to fight infection and promote healing. It can help prevent illness and keep your immune system strong when taken daily.

Tips

Always check with your doctor before using any substitute for medication. In addition to this herbal drink remedy, addressing issues that lower your immune system, like stress, is crucial. Remember, vitamin D is essential to boost immunity and increase your ability to fight against sickness.

If you don't have all of the ingredients on hand, you can omit those you don't have. This remedy can also be made with fresh ginger and garlic if desired.

Caution

This herbal drink remedy is not for everyone. Do not take this herbal drink remedy if you are pregnant or breastfeeding. Compared to conventional antibiotics, this remedy has fewer side effects. If you have any medical condition, please consult your doctor before taking this herbal drink.

Usnea Tincture

Usnea is a lichen that has been used medicinally for centuries. It is a powerful antibacterial, antiviral, and antifungal agent. Usnea can be used internally and externally.

Ingredients:
- 1 ounce of dried usnea
- 1 pint of vodka or other high-proof alcohol

Instructions:
1. Combine the usnea and alcohol in a glass jar and seal tightly.
2. Store the jar in a dark, cool place for four to six weeks, shaking it daily to help release the usnic acid from the plant material.
3. After four to six weeks, strain the liquid through a coffee filter or piece of cheesecloth and store it in a dark glass bottle.
4. Take one teaspoon of tincture two to three times daily.

Benefit

Usnea is a potent herbal antibiotic used to treat various infections. It is especially effective against gram-positive bacteria like staphylococcus and streptococcus. Usnea can also help fight viral and fungal infections.

Usnea tincture can be used in various ways to treat different ailments. When used externally, it helps speed up the healing of cuts and scrapes while also preventing infection. It can be taken internally to treat respiratory infections, urinary tract infections, and stomach viruses. It also benefits those wanting to lose weight and have sore throats.

Tips

If you are using usnea tincture internally, shake the bottle well before each dose. Usnea tincture can be taken for long periods without any adverse effects.

Usnea tincture can be taken internally by adding 1-2 drops to a glass of water or juice or used topically by adding a few drops to a cotton ball and applying it to the affected area. Usnea tincture can also be added to homemade cleaning solutions to boost disinfection power.

Caution

Usnea is powerful medicine and should be used with caution if you are pregnant or breastfeeding. If you have allergies to plants in the Parmeliaceae family (including usnea), you should not take this herb. As with any herbal remedy, it is always best to consult a healthcare professional before taking a usnea tincture or other herbal remedy.

Herbal Tea for Cough Relief

This herbal tea recipe is a great way to soothe a cough naturally. The tea is made with only a few simple ingredients and can be taken as needed.

Ingredients:

- 1 teaspoon of dried peppermint leaves
- 1 teaspoon of dried chamomile flowers
- 1 teaspoon of honey
- 1 cup of boiling water

Instructions:

1. Mix the chamomile flowers, peppermint leaves, and honey into a mug.
2. Pour boiling water over the ingredients and allow to steep for 5-10 minutes.
3. Strain the tea and drink as needed.

Benefits

Peppermint is an excellent herb for relieving coughing and congestion. Chamomile is also helpful in soothing coughs and easing anxiety. Honey is a natural cough suppressant and helps coat the throat.

Tips

You can use fresh mint leaves if you don't have dried peppermint leaves but increase the steeping time to 10 minutes.

Caution

This tea is not suitable for children under the age of 12. If you are pregnant or breastfeeding, please consult your doctor before drinking this tea.

The recipes in the book are a great way to start using herbal antibiotics. They are easy to make and don't require fancy equipment. They help fight infection if used correctly, even if they are not as powerful as prescription antibiotics.

However, it is essential to remember that these remedies should preferably be used at the onset of illness. You should always consult your doctor before taking any medication, including herbal antibiotics.

Mother Nature kindly offers these herbs for our benefit. They are readily available in most stores or online. Better yet, grow your own and educate yourself and your family on the many features and benefits that herbs offer.

Remember, before consuming or using herbs, research or read books and guides to determine if they would suit your purpose.

Conclusion

While incredibly helpful in acute infections, the overuse of synthetic antibiotics has caused them to be less and less effective. In recent years, more and more strains of antibiotic-resistant bacteria have developed because people use antibiotics without being aware of their full effects. These strains resist the effects of antibiotics, which adversely affect a patient's body. It destroys the gut microbiome, overloads the liver, and, in large doses, damages the kidneys.

Herbal antibiotics carry fewer of these effects. They're also more effective in killing the bacteria causing the infection. Herbal antibiotics have a slightly different way of acting in your body, and the bacteria are less likely to resist them. Herbal antibiotics made from natural ingredients are particularly recommended to those who want to avoid the effects of preservatives and other additives used in artificial drugs. Whether you've experienced the negative effects of these ingredients or currently taking other medications and don't want to risk cross-reactivity, you'll benefit from herbal antibiotics. Herbal antibiotics are an excellent alternative for treating common ailments, even if you merely want to ensure you get the maximum benefits.

You must choose between systemic, non-systemic, and synergetic antibiotics depending on the condition being treated. Systemic antibiotics act on a systemic level, traveling through the bloodstream toward all body parts. Non-systemic antibiotics have a localized effect. Due to their size, they are not easily transmitted to cell membranes. Lastly, synergetic herbs facilitate the action of other antibiotics or medicine in several ways, including guiding the medicine molecules to the right place or allowing them to bond with the appropriate receptors.

However, you must remember that the primary function is to kill bacteria, even those in your gut and skin; these are part of your body's natural defense mechanism. Herbal antibiotics carry fewer risks as they are more effective, and you won't need to use them as long as you would synthetic ones. However, their prolonged use still leads to a weakened immune system. Therefore, use other natural medicine that restores the balance of healthy bacterial growth in your body to build immunity. Restoring the microbiome will also avoid other symptoms like diarrhea and digestion issues that further deplete your body's reserves. This allows your immune system to catch any imbalance the next time harmful bacteria attack you.

Once you learn about the benefits of using herbal antivirals, you're ready to move on to making them. This book taught you which tools you need to prepare natural medicine and grow your own herbs. The latter is particularly recommended if you want to ensure using organic ingredients. After mastering the skills needed to grow and harvest your plants, you can incorporate them into the recipes provided in the last two chapters. They're accompanied by a thorough explanation of how the specific combination of ingredients will make you feel better. You'll be prepared to treat each common condition with the appropriate antibiotics.

References

Sengupta, S., Chattopadhyay, M. K., & Grossart, H.-P. (2013). The multifaceted roles of antibiotics and antibiotic resistance in nature. Frontiers in Microbiology, 4, 47. https://doi.org/10.3389/fmicb.2013.00047

Antibiotics. (1999). Drug Therapy. https://medlineplus.gov/antibiotics.html

Antibiotics. (n.d.). EMedicineHealth. https://www.emedicinehealth.com/antibiotics/article_em.htm

7 best natural antibiotics: Uses, evidence, and effectiveness. (2020, January 1). Medicalnewstoday.com. https://www.medicalnewstoday.com/articles/321108

Pancu, D. F., Scurtu, A., Macasoi, I. G., Marti, D., Mioc, M., Soica, C., Coricovac, D., Horhat, D., Poenaru, M., & Dehelean, C. (2021). Antibiotics: Conventional therapy and natural compounds with antibacterial activity-A pharmaco-toxicological screening. Antibiotics (Basel, Switzerland), 10(4), 401. https://doi.org/10.3390/antibiotics10040401

Brusie, C. (2016, November 23). What are the most effective natural antibiotics? Healthline. https://www.healthline.com/health/natural-antibiotics

Jillian Levy, C. (2021, September 21). 15 fermented foods for a healthy gut and overall health. Dr. Axe. https://draxe.com/nutrition/fermented-foods/

Kris Gunnars, B. (2022, May 27). 5 health benefits of apple cider vinegar.

Van De Walle, G., MS, & RD. (2019, February 11). Pau D'Arco: Uses, benefits, side effects, and dosage. Healthline. https://www.healthline.com/nutrition/pau-d-arco

PAU D'ARCO: Overview, uses, side effects, precautions, interactions, dosing, and reviews. (n.d.). Webmd.com. https://www.webmd.com/vitamins/ai/ingredientmono-647/pau-darco

Landsiedel, K. (n.d.). Dobson Bay Chiropractic. Dobsonbaychiro.com https://www.dobsonbaychiro.com/blogs/natural-antibiotics.html

GOLDENSEAL: Overview, uses, side effects, precautions, interactions, dosing, and reviews. (n.d.). Webmd.com. https://www.webmd.com/vitamins/ai/ingredientmono-943/goldenseal

Link, R., MS, & RD. (2020, March 12). 8 surprising health benefits of cloves. Healthline. https://www.healthline.com/nutrition/benefits-of-cloves

Herbal alternatives to antibiotics. (2021, January 26). Mother Earth Living - Healthy Life, Natural Beauty. https://www.motherearthliving.com/health-and-wellness/alternatives-to-antibiotics-zm0z12aszdeb/

Lee, S.-Y., Kwon, H.-K., & Lee, S.-M. (2011). SHINBARO, a new herbal medicine with a multifunctional mechanism for joint disease: first therapeutic application for the treatment of osteoarthritis. Archives of Pharmacal Research, 34(11), 1773–1777. https://doi.org/10.1007/s12272-011-1121-0

7 best natural antibiotics: Uses, evidence, and effectiveness. (2020, January 1). Medicalnewstoday.com. https://www.medicalnewstoday.com/articles/321108

GOLDENSEAL: Overview, uses, side effects, precautions, interactions, dosing, and reviews. (n.d.). Webmd.com. from https://www.webmd.com/vitamins/ai/ingredientmono-943/goldenseal

Neverman, L. (2020, November 27). Herbal antibiotics - using herbs to fight infection and speed healing. Common Sense Home; Common Sense Home LLC. https://commonsensehome.com/herbal-antibiotics/

Antibiotic-resistant bacteria. (n.d.). Gov.au. https://www.betterhealth.vic.gov.au/health/conditionsandtreatments/antibiotic-resistant-bacteria

Kuok, C.-F., Hoi, S.-O., Hoi, C.-F., Chan, C.-H., Fong, I.-H., Ngok, C.-K., Meng, L.-R., & Fong, P. (2017). Synergistic antibacterial effects of herbal extracts and antibiotics on methicillin-resistant Staphylococcus aureus: A computational and experimental study. Experimental Biology and Medicine (Maywood, N.J.), 242(7), 731–743. https://doi.org/10.1177/1535370216689828

Torella, J. P., Chait, R., & Kishony, R. (2010). Optimal drug synergy in antimicrobial treatments. PLoS Computational Biology, 6(6), e1000796. https://doi.org/10.1371/journal.pcbi.1000796

7 best natural antibiotics: Uses, evidence, and effectiveness. (2020, January 1). Medicalnewstoday.com. https://www.medicalnewstoday.com/articles/321108

Antibiotic resistance. (n.d.-a). Who. int. https://www.who.int/news-room/fact-sheets/detail/antibiotic-resistance

Antibiotic resistance. (n.d.-b). Nhs. uk. https://www.nhs.uk/conditions/antibiotics/antibiotic-antimicrobial-resistance/

Brusie, C. (2016, November 23). What are the most effective natural antibiotics? Healthline. https://www.healthline.com/health/natural-antibiotics

Landsiedel, K. (n.d.). Dobson Bay Chiropractic. Dobsonbaychiro.com. https://www.dobsonbaychiro.com/blogs/natural-antibiotics.html

McCallum, K. (n.d.). 6 ways to boost your immune system. Houstonmethodist.org. https://www.houstonmethodist.org/blog/articles/2020/mar/5-ways-to-boost-your-immune-system/

Shoemaker, S., MS, RDN, & LD. (2020, April 1). 9 tips to strengthen your immunity naturally. Healthline. https://www.healthline.com/nutrition/how-to-boost-immune-health

Gilmer, M. (2020, April 13). Strengthen your immune system with 4 simple strategies. Cleveland Clinic. https://health.clevelandclinic.org/strengthen-your-immune-system-with-simple-strategies/

Yang, S. (2021, January 16). 20 herbs that can boost your immune system. The Thirty. https://thethirty.whowhatwear.com/herbs-to-boost-immune-system/slide23

Svedi, R. (2007, March 11). Top ten herb garden benefits. Gardening Know How. https://www.gardeningknowhow.com/edible/herbs/hgen/the-top-ten-benefits-of-growing-your-own-herb-garden.htm

Kilbride, B. (n.d.). Gardening tools we consider indispensable: It doesn't take much! Almanac.com. https://www.almanac.com/gardening-tools-guide

Zhang, J., Onakpoya, I. J., Posadzki, P., & Eddouks, M. (2015). The safety of herbal medicine: from prejudice to evidence. Evidence-Based Complementary and Alternative Medicine: ECAM, 2015, 316706. https://doi.org/10.1155/2015/316706

No title. (n.d.). Lancastergeneralhealth.org. https://lancastergeneralhealth.org/health-hub-home/2021/june/5-reasons-to-be-cautious-when-considering-herbal-remedies

Lang, A., BSc, MBA, & Scaccia, A. (2020, April 13). How to peel: Ginger.

THYME: Overview, uses, side effects, precautions, interactions, dosing, and reviews. (n.d.). Webmd.com. https://www.webmd.com/vitamins/ai/ingredientmono-823/thyme

Lemon balm tea: Types, benefits, and more. (2022, February 4). Medicalnewstoday.com. https://www.medicalnewstoday.com/articles/lemon-balm-tea

Brusie, C. (2016, November 23). What are the most effective natural antibiotics? Healthline. https://www.healthline.com/health/natural-antibiotics

www.ingramcontent.com/pod-product-compliance
Lightning Source LLC
LaVergne TN
LVHW021817060526
838201LV00058B/3423